MW00570007

Another BAG Another DAY

Creating a new Lease on Life in a New World

by
Jo-Ann L. Tremblay

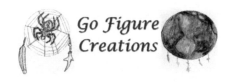

Ottawa Canada
Go Figure Creations
www.jo-annltremblay.com
Blog: joannltremblay.wordpress.com
facebook: Jo-Ann L. Tremblay
Twitter: @joanntremblay

Copyright © 2015 Jo-Ann L. Tremblay

1st Edition

All rights reserved. No part of this book may be reproduced or transmitted in any form or by any means, electronic or mechanical, including photocopying, recording, electronic transmission, or by any storage and retrieval system, without the prior written permission from the author or the publisher.

First Go Figure Creations electronic edition September 23, 2015

Amazon.com edition September 23, 2015

Designed by Go Figure Creations

Cover design copyright © 2015 Go Figure Creations

Cover Photo copyright © 2015 Jo-Ann L. Tremblay

Author's Photo by Mark J. R. Henderson

ISBN-13: 978-0-9809009-2-7

DEDICATION

Mark, thank you for sharing life with Percy and me. We're having the time of our lives.

Richard, thank you for your strength and courage.

Thank you to the children and grandchildren of our blended family, you're the best.

Thank you for all who have come before me, my patriarchs and matriarchs, you are all an inspiration.

In addition, this book is dedicated to all who have and will have an ostomy, and to the families, friends, caregivers, and medical professionals, who will join them on their journey to their new normal, their new world.

Table of Contents

Table of Contents

Table of Contents

Table of Contents

Table of Contents

Prologue

It's been a year and a day since Percy Stoma was created. I'm an ostomate and without Percy I would not have the opportunity to live my second chance at life.

You keep me alive, thanks little buddy.

You're welcome Jo-Ann.

Together as a team we're working hard to recover and adjust to our new normal, and deep in my bones I feel something profound is happening. The underlying message of this feeling is; the anticipation that something great or something terrible is happening. Within this confusion lies the adventure of the life and healing journey. How much recovery will actually occur? Is there a limit or is it limitless?

The healing journey continues ...

PART 1

Losing Myself

1.0 Introduction

Knock, knock.
Who's there?
Osto.
Osto who?
The ostomanator. Aha. It's all in the bag now!

Oh Percy, hold on, we're not there yet, we're just getting started. There's no doubt, life with you is a second chance at life, the icing on the cake with a cherry on top. We've come a long way since our lifesaving surgery July 21, 2011 when you were created. And it's been a long — at times hard but mostly amazing — journey to date. Percy, that was a cute joke, but let's not get ahead of ourselves.

Hello dear reader, my name is Jo-Ann L. Tremblay. I'm an ostomate and author of *Better WITH a Bag Than IN a Bag*, a book that chronicles my devastating illness, emergency lifesaving surgery, the creation of Percy (my stoma), and the year-long recovery that brought me to my first stomaversary. On that day, we enjoyed a celebration of life with friends, good eats and all the sparkle July 21, 2012 could bring. On July 22, 2012, the following day, the full impact of reality set in and I realized that although the official recovery period was now completed, the lingering damage from the original disease, the damage from the extensive surgery and the emotional toll it takes to adapt and live with an altered body function was just beginning. Percy, my life-sustaining stoma and I are at the beginning of our "beginning again". Hmm ... well, ah ... at the beginning of the what, who, when, where, and how of a new life, a new self and a new normal, whatever the heck it's all supposed to be.

So many changes occur for anyone and everyone when they must face illness, a significant emotional event, or life alteration(s), whether chosen or thrust upon them. Often feeling trapped by life's condition, people experience a form of the grieving process. Research tells us the process goes like this: 1. Shock and denial, 2. Pain and guilt, 3. Anger and bargaining, 4. Depression, reflection, and loneliness, 5. The upward turn, 6. Reconstruction and working through, 7. Acceptance and hope. We will experience these stages not necessarily one after the other, instead, we feel any one of them at any given time and sometimes, we feel all of them at the same time.

Ostomates such as I are not an exception. So to boil it down, the process from an ostomate's prospective that we experience is:

Shock: Numbness, Why me?

Denial: It's not me.

This is not happening.

Bargaining: I'll try anything.

Anger: If only the doctor were better,

Blame family/job.

Depression: I'm damaged goods.

Nothing will be OK again.

Acceptance: I'll do the best I can. Self-Care

One of the keys to successfully navigating our path is to know and believe time does not heal. Instead, know that it takes time and work to heal the body, mind, emotions and the human spirit.

Marching forward to the beat of the recovery drum that sets the pace is what this book is about. Regardless of your life-altering occurrence, the truth and authenticity of whatever has struck you like a bolt of lightning cannot be erased. The next key to successfully navigating your life is to know and believe that grief is not a place where we stand stuck, it's a process, a challenging and remarkable journey.

Join me and my clever stoma, Percy, as we commit to living a joyous and full life, weave our tapestry of human experience, and learn to work together as a team.

Let's face it, living is not for wimps and none of us can change the past. We cannot take away or erase the incident(s) or the circumstance(s) that started everything. What we can do is put one foot in front of the other, continue on our way in spite of it all and accept come what may.

Why have Percy and I invited you to read this book, and navigate through the journey together? Because no person can fix us as individuals but our own selves. The people in our lives can do something(s) but they really — in the final analysis — cannot fully do anything in particular. What we most need is to know we are cared for and supported. The rest is all up to us individually.

Every day, every one of us has another chance at life. It's the icing on the cake with the cherry on top. This book is my individualized true story and how I perceived it. It's an ordinary woman's story in many ways but although the circumstances will vary, it is everyone's life story. I truly believe that everyone we meet has a story to tell! I know I can knock on any door, anywhere on planet Earth, and it will be answered by a person who has endured something(s), and is working to make himself and his life work out to the best of his abilities. The healing journey continues ...

1.1 Disconnected and Frayed

A number of years ago, I read an ancient story. As I recall, it goes something like this: A monk hoists a yoke onto his shoulders. Hanging from each side of the yoke is an empty bucket. Everyday he walks down the mountain path till he reaches the pond below. He dips the buckets into the clear water and fills them. Then, with the buckets filled, he trudges back up the mountain path. At the top, he empties the buckets into a container then, once again, he walks back down the mountain path. He dips his buckets in, fills them, then trudges back up the mountain, empties the buckets, walks down the path, and so on. One day, he reaches the top of the mountain and this time he becomes filled with enlightenment. He experiences the *OM*'s and *aha*'s of a truly inspirational enlightened moment. Then, he hoists the yoke back onto his shoulders, walks down the mountain, dips his buckets in, fills the buckets, trudges up the mountain, empties the buckets, and then returns back down the mountain ... The moral of the story as I understand it is: Before enlightenment there is chopping wood and carrying water. After enlightenment there is chopping wood and carrying water. In other words, life is what it is. From time to time there are sprinkles of amazing shifts from dark to light and then, life continues to be what it is, yet forever changed.

At this point, I can really relate to the monk. My life is saved. Wow. Amazing. How enlightening this is! I poop in a bag. Oh my, really? I'm doing my best to tote my recovery and ostomy buckets all the while feeling it's raining on me even when the sun is shining.

Oops ... I think this is another fine occasion to organize a pity party and Percy you're my invited guest.

As I climb life's mountain, Percy is now prolapsed, my parastomal hernia is growing larger by the day , and the profile from the left side of my abdomen is that of a five-month expectant mother while the right side of my abdomen is relatively un-pregnant looking. Talk about a major wedgie! Geez, there isn't a piece of clothing that fits me comfortably, starting with my underwear. (For more information on prolapsed stoma and parastomal hernia, go to "Information, Tips & Hints" section.)

I sure don't feel normal as I try to launch and immerse myself into my new normal. How ridiculous *new normal* sounds to me, right now.

To add to my, um ... joy, I'm now addressing tissue, organ and nerve damage resulting from the original disease (diverticular disease). For four long years this disease resulted in serious infections on an ongoing basis, infections that remained improperly diagnosed. During this time, the ravages of the disease caused the development of multiple bowel perforations. The perforations allowed toxins — including excrement — to leak into my abdominal cavity. As I was told, if I had arrived at the hospital an hour later on that fateful day, I most probably would not have survived. The surgeon, Dr.

Auer, suggested to my husband, Mark, that we should say our goodbyes before I was wheeled into the operating theatre as my chances for survival were pretty low. I was almost sent back to the stars.

How marvellous when you really think about it, after what was finally an accurate diagnosis by the emergency department doctor and team at the General Hospital, Ottawa, Canada that, in just short of eight hours, a team of eight specialists repaired damage, created my stoma, and essentially carved me into a survivor. I am forever grateful to these amazing doctors, nurses and my caregiver (Mark), who were with me all the way through the darkest hours. Now I realize, though, that this was not only my "beginning again", but it really was just the "beginning" of what would turn out to be a horrible and amazing journey called "recovery" — recovery that includes not only physical healing, but emotional, mental and human-spirit repair, as well.

The reality I face at this time is that I sustained extensive nerve damage to my lower spine, vagina and urethra, and those are the apparent victims of both the ravages of the disease and the invasive lifesaving surgery. It has always been all-or-nothing for me in my life, but the totality of this reality really does seem extreme, even for me, for goodness sake.

Deja poo, Jo-Ann!

Excuse me, Percy. For goodness sake, what do you mean?

Well, you're facing another major surgery.

Yes, you're right. Another major surgery is in the future. This one is to repair my parastomal hernia and to insert a bio mesh, which includes putting you, Percy, into a supportive mesh hammock. It's scheduled for ... Well. Let's see. October, November of 2012, January, February of 2013, oh and let's just say sometime during the spring of 2013. I'm sitting here waiting to hear from my surgeon's assistant in the next while ... hmm ... well, sometime ...

"I recommend that you don't wait by the phone," she advises. "We'll get back to you in the next while."

Meanwhile, I look in horror at my ever-widening abdominal horizons. Like an old string of Christmas lights that were stored away haphazardly last year, I'm a jumble of tangled wires. I am all knotted up and I just want to stay rolled up in a ball. I'm literally and figuratively a bundle of disconnected and frayed nerves and this is affecting me physically and emotionally, not to mention how low my mental state and my human spirit are sinking to.

I feel my light needs to sparkle and shine once again. I want to be light and life. I do have high hopes. But, before this can happen I have to unknot, unravel and straighten myself out. I have to recover, but how much recovery will actually occur? Is there a limit, or is it limitless?

1.2 Battlefields of the Body

Although the nerve damage to my body parts are seriously affecting me in many ways, at the same time I am excited. I'm enthusiastic because for the first time in a number of years, I'm not waking up during the night to void. At my age, this is fantastic. Sweet whole nights of sleep. Wonderful dreamtime nights with no multiple trips to the bathroom. Full nights of uninterrupted, blissful sleep. Happy, happy, skippy skippy. But after a few weeks I realized, even when I woke up in the morning after a full night's sleep, although I know I have a full bladder, I still don't feel the urge to urinate. Hold on a minute here, this isn't right.

When I do attempt, well let's just say that things are just not flowing for me. Oh, dear. It's time to make another visit to my Internal Specialist, Dr. Onochie, yet again. He is my Santa Claus, my Earth Angel, the very doctor who took the time to listen to me in June of 2011 before everything fell apart in my body and I underwent the *colectomy* and my ostomy was created. He's the doctor who worked fervently to pull together the healing team of five, and the one who had assured me that he and the team would do everything to figure things out. He was the doctor who listened to me when others wouldn't, and he expected me to be a part of my own healing team. He gave me hope in that June. Blessed hope, and it was wonderful.

Sitting in the chair in his office, I once again looked into his big brown eyes, as I explained my concerns. After a moment of quiet thought he stated, "You're correct, this isn't right. I'm referring you to a urologist. Don't worry, we'll figure this out," he assured me. Oh, how I remember those words *we'll figure this out* uttered by him a year and a bit ago. Leaving his office, I feel more confident, and once again I'm left with a feeling of hope.

Meanwhile, I am facing another major surgery in three, four, six or whatever months from now. It's only been just over a year since my last major surgery and I know it is time to take a good hard look at myself to ascertain what physical shape I'm in as I prepare for the next round. Time to educate myself on foods and other lifestyle additions that I can use to give me the best crack at surviving through, then recovering from, the upcoming surgery. I'm ready to take the reins in both hands, to be the best I can be.

Optimism rules the day as I make an appointment with my skilful and enthusiastic physiotherapist, Dr. Sarah Cohen — Dynamic Ottawa, to work with me. Our intent is to develop an exercise program to build up my body and to prepare me for the surgery. Filled with the spark of eagerness that I'm getting a head start, I arrived for my appointment.

Before we began, she instructed me to board the walking treadmill and walk for a few minutes. Climbing onto the machine, I imagine with each step I take that I'm planting my footprints, I'm journeying with the intent of going beyond striving, to arrive at thriving.

Sarah's knowledge of kinesiology and her professional know-how are exceptional. I have the utmost respect and confidence in her ability to bring her skills, ideas, health background and enthusiasm to each client in need, which includes me. After a few minutes on the treadmill, she walked up beside the machine and instructed me to keep walking. "You've got drop foot," she said.

I turned the machine off, looked down at my feet, and struggled to hold back my tears. I don't know what drop foot is but it sure doesn't sound good to me. Whatever this is, I instinctively know on top of everything, I am going to have to face another struggle. I've been spending the last number of years keeping my head above the waves, and in an instant, I feel myself being dragged down into the depths of despair, yet again. (For more information on drop foot, go to the "Information, Tips & Hints" section.)

Is this my new life, my new me? I poop in a bag, for goodness sake, my abdomen is a lopsided bulge, I can't pee properly, and now my foot is dropping. Some track I'm on. Well, that's it isn't it. I am on a track, just like the one I'm standing on right now. I'm working hard at putting one foot ahead of the other, trying to get somewhere and, frankly, I don't seem to be getting anywhere. Must admit, a nasty thought flashed through my mind in that moment. Without being too graphic, I imagined ripping Percy Stoma's bag off and pitching it. I envisioned it arcing over Sarah's head as it executed a one and a half gainer, a gainer because I'm an artist and I think this is a creative touch. Then it sails through the air, zinging past the exercise equipment to smash onto the far wall. Needless to say, I've seen better days.

Immediately following this vision, the wisdom of my dear Granny came to mind. She had taught me at the age of 4, "A man of words and not of deeds is like a garden full of weeds." Not sure why this thought came to mind in that moment. The vision of Percy's bag and a brown mess smashed on a wall was certainly not a deed my Granny had in mind when she taught it to me. I know there is a nugget of wisdom waiting for me just below the surface here, but I'm going to need some time to mine my emotions, my mind, and my human spirit to find it.

1.3 Percy Toots His Own Horn

Whoa Jo-Ann. Press the pause button. Not everyone experiences the same issues we're dealing with right now. In fact, not everyone has a colostomy, either. There's a lot of stomas I have met who are quite different than me.

You're right, Percy. Thanks for reminding me.

Percy is absolutely correct in mentioning we have our differences. Let's go back to basics for a moment. We as humans have a small intestine, a large intestine and a urinary tract.

Small Intestine

The small intestine runs from the stomach to the large intestine and has three main sections; the duodenum, which is the first ten inches; the jejunum, which is the middle eight feet; and the ileum, which is the final twelve feet. It extends to the ileocecal valve, which empties into the colon (large intestine). The ileum is suspended from the abdominal wall by the mesentery, a fold of serous (moisture-secreting) membrane.

Large Intestine

The large intestine is about five feet long and runs from the small intestine to the anus. The colon and rectum are the two main sections of the large intestine. Semisolid digestive waste enters the colon from the small intestine. Gradually, the colon absorbs moisture and forms stool as digestive waste moves toward the rectum. The rectum is about six inches long and is located right before the anus. The rectum stores stool. The rectum and anus control bowel movements.

Stoma

Certain diseases of the bowel or urinary tract involve removing all or part of the intestine or bladder. This creates a need for an alternate way for feces or urine to leave the body. An opening is surgically created in the abdomen for body waste to pass through. The surgical procedure is called an ostomy. The opening that is created at the end of the bowel or ureter is called a stoma, which is pulled through the abdominal wall.

Several Surgical Options Exist For Bowel Diversion

An *ileostomy* diverts the ileum to a stoma. An ileostomy bypasses the colon, rectum, and anus. The waste flows out of the stoma and collects in an ostomy bag.

A *colostomy* is similar to an ileostomy, but the colon — not the ileum is diverted to a stoma. As with an ileostomy, stool collects in an ostomy bag.

Hey, that's me, I'm a colostomy!

Yes, Percy, you sure are.

Ileoanal reservoir surgery is an option when the large intestine is removed but the anus remains intact and disease-free. The surgeon creates a colon-like pouch called an ileoanal reservoir, from the last several inches of the ileum. The ileoanal reservoir is also called a **pelvic** or **J-pouch**. Stool collects in the ileoanal reservoir that exits the body through the anus as a bowel movement. In the case of a J-pouch, there are usually two or more surgeries required, including a temporary ileostomy. An adjustment period lasting several months is needed for the newly formed ileoanal reservoir to stretch and adjust to its new function.

A **urostomy** is a surgical procedure that diverts urine away from a diseased or defective bladder. Among several methods to create the urostomy, the most common method at the time of this book's printing, is usually referred to as the Bricker Ileal Conduit, after its inventor, Eugene M. Bricker. Either a section at the end of the small intestine (ileum) or at the beginning of the large intestine (cecum) is relocated surgically to form a stoma for urine to pass out of the body. Other common names for this procedure are **ileal loop** or **colon conduit**.

A urostomy may be performed due to bladder cancer, spinal cord injuries, malfunction of the bladder, or due to birth defects such as spina bifida.

Since colostomy, ileostomy, and urostomy bypass the sphincter muscle, there is no voluntary control over bowel/urine movements. All ostomies require an external pouch that must be worn to catch the discharge.

Some people need only a temporary bowel diversion; others need a permanent bowel diversion.

There are many reasons why a person would need a bowel diversion. The most common are: cancer, trauma, inflammatory bowel diseases (IBD), diverticular disease, Chron's, bowel obstruction, and diverticulitis, to name a few.

People who undergo bowel diversion surgery range from the newborn to the elderly, and every age in between.

There are many other types of bowel diversions and ostomies. For more information go to: www.ostomycanada.ca

I'll hand this next part over to you, Percy.

I know you like to toot your own horn, Percy. In fact, you toot it any time and anywhere, interrupting as you please. You know it can be rather embarrassing.

Sorry. You know I just can't control myself, it all just comes spilling out.

Yes, well, Percy. I think it's a good time to go back and share some history with our readers. Take it away Percy.

Ah, hmm .... I'd like to start with a bit of history. Creations such as myself have been around for quite some time now. The word stoma is derived from Greek — for mouth or opening. Jo-Ann and Mark (her husband and caregiver) named me Percy. Percy name origin: old English for "pierce the hedge". How brilliant is that? By the way, they did not name me to be cute in any way. I was given my name to be used as a code word. For example, if we're out and Jo-Ann is having some issues with me and knows she may end up spending a while in a bathroom due to me requiring a change of equipment, all she has to say to Mark is "Percy needs attention." Mark then knows not to be concerned if she takes longer than usual in the facility. My code name is useful in many other circumstances and situations, as well.

It's purported that the ancient Greeks speculated about the role of surgical intervention for intestinal obstruction. Ancient Greek physicians such as Hippocrates (460–377 BC) and Celsus (53BC–7 AD) wrote that wounds of the large intestine need not be deadly, whereas wounds of the small intestine and bladder were.

Another ancient medical figure was Galen (130–200 AD) who was a surgeon to Emperor Marcus Aurelius and the Roman gladiators. In his writings, he discussed surgical management of the large intestine and abdominal wall following penetrating injuries; however, it is understood that he believed little could be done to save the person with a rupture of the small intestine.

Not until the eighteenth century did intentional ostomy surgery occur. In our research, the first recorded Royal to have an ostomy was Queen Caroline (wife of George II) who died on November 20, 1737, days after the surgery — her strangulated bowel burst — at St. James's Palace. The first planned stoma was created in 1776, and the credit goes to M. Pillore, a French surgeon who operated on M. Morel. *Vive la France!*

The first successful colostomy recorded was performed by a French surgeon, Duret, in 1793 on an infant who was born without a rectum. Although the infant was close to death prior to surgery, he recovered to live for 45 more years. Throughout the remainder of the eighteenth century, contributions from others led to the acceptance of surgical intervention for refractory intestinal obstruction.

The first recorded operative ileostomy was in 1879 by Baum, a German surgeon from Danzig. A temporary ileostomy was performed on a patient with a malignant obstruction; however, the patient died just over nine weeks later from peritonitis. A successful recovery in a patient following an ileostomy procedure was reported by Maydi from Vienna in 1883.

Ileostomies carried with them unacceptably high mortality rates up until the 1950s. As it turns out, successful urinary diversions were not achieved until the 1950s either, when an American surgeon, Eugene Bricker, described a new procedure, and since the 1950s, Bricker's ileal conduit procedure has remained the most commonly used technique for urinary diversion.

It was in the 1950s that physicians contributed greatly to the understanding of stoma physiology. It was also at this time it was recognized that there was a need to develop specialists in ostomy care. And so, with the assistance of patients, the first school for Enterostomal Therapists (ET) opened.

Advances in stoma therapy and surgical management have made it possible for millions of individuals with stomas, worldwide, with the ability to maintain a close-to-normal lifestyle.

We stomas are amazing creations, if I may say so myself, and some of us are famous. We have actively engaged on the battlefield, stood before the masses on stage in theatres, our contributions to our community of humanity are many. We are actors, dancers, sports stars; we're on television, and more.

Some of our members of the *fellowship of the bag* are:

Fred Astaire — actor/dancer

Frank Sinatra — November 9, 1986 — reversal January 1987

Rolf Joachim Benirschke — professional US football player

Napoleon Bonaparte — world leader/military conqueror

Pope John Paul II — had an ostomy in 1981 following an assassination attempt — reversal August 1981

Marvin Bush — financial advisor and son of former US President

Al Geiberger — professional golfer

Bob Hope — entertainer/comedian/actor

Tip O'Neil — US Speaker of the House and Ambassador to Ireland

Queen Mum — British Royal

Ed Sullivan — TV host

Loretta Young — actress

Thank you Percy for the historical back story. I hear you shouting (or in your case, tooting) a bravo for the people who, no matter their challenges, have searched, discovered and gotten on with life in spite of it all. Hmm ... I guess I'm not

really there yet. Time to flip my eyes inward and take a good long look at where I'm at.

1.4 Battlefields of the Body — Part Two

Arriving at the brink of death and surviving against the odds was an amazing triumph of the surgical medical team, home-care workers, my caregiver, Mark, and my body and human spirit. I fully embrace the full and glorious extent of this. I am in awe.

I had spent the following year after the surgery on the battlefield of recovery. My goal was to transform myself through a spectacular recovery. What I didn't account for at the time was that there would be so much long-term damage from the original disease. I did not realize what would be the added physical carnage due to the length of time it had taken the attending physicians to diagnose my medical condition prior to that fateful day. I was clueless of the extent of destruction a surgery of this kind could have on a body. The attack on my body due to the various potent medications that had been pumped *intravenously* into me, and that I also had to consume orally both before and after the surgery, was unknown to me.

I know that sometimes when something bad happens, we think if we wait long enough it will all go away. Well, as life would have it, nothing was going away. In fact, things are being added to my challenge list:

I poop in a bag

I have a parastomal hernia

I have a prolapsed stoma

I can't pee properly

I have drop foot

I must prepare my body, mind and spirit for another major surgery

And, the newest addition:

Medication-induced psoriasis (on my hands, heels, and the bottom of my feet)

I'm at the beginning of the what, who, when, where and how of my new self and life, my new normal, whatever the heck that's all supposed to be. I'm human and what happened to me has caused me to endure the grieving process, yet again, in this life experience. Taking stock of myself with each added item on my challenge list at this juncture, I really feel I'm experiencing the first 4 stages of grief all at the same time. Each new challenging item is shocking me and I sure would like to indulge in denial. I'm in pain. I'm angry. And if I could bargain myself out of this fix, you can bet your bottom dollar I would.

I'm reflecting now, I don't feel depressed but I sure am profoundly sad. I need to be conscious of and work on the #5 to #7 stages (5. The upward turn; 6. Reconstruction and working through) of the grieving process and get on with my upward turn, which is acceptance and the hope that's the #7 stage of this annoying process.

Looking back (reflection, that's the #4 stage), my son Richard drifts into my inner vision. This darling little fella was born with deformed/crooked hips, legs and feet. Most of us stand with the toes of our feet facing one and the same direction. My son stood toe to toe. One foot faced inward left and the other foot and toes faced inward right.

There were years of on-and-off casts and braces on his legs. Physiotherapy, orthopaedic shoes and so on. There were panels of doctors who advised us he would never walk properly. He would never be able to run, skate, and the list went on. We decided that our son would lead the way. We would do anything and everything necessary, and we would use our own creativity to assist him. It was not just his body we parented, it was also his emotions, intellect and human spirit. We never told him he could or would not walk, run, climb, and so on. We simply urged him on, and with every wobbly step he took, we celebrated his accomplishments with no expectations, or any limits.

The wisest advice we received at that time was not to run and pick him up when he fell. Not to, within reason of course, rescue or coddle him. But I must admit I felt sad and worried for him. Life is hard enough as it is and my son had added mobility challenges.

At a year and a half old, when the first sets of casts and braces were removed, he stood up on his tangled feet and proceeded to make his way across the living room. This was his first time, and I observed him with pride and joy in my heart. We clapped and squealed in delight together, we both felt on top of the world!

During this adventure across the living room, I had also observed him bump into, and get winged by furniture as he banged into everything in his path, and then he smashed into the far wall. It was as though he didn't see them. He had literally gone from Point A to Point B, hitting everything along the way, and he didn't even seem to realize he was at Point B, until he went splat right into it.

Okay, his hips, legs and feet don't work well, but the little fella didn't seem to be aware of the obstacles in the room. Until that time, he had only been able to crawl using his arms like a soldier in combat due to the casts. Of course this was at a much slower pace than walking, and at other times, we had carried him or pushed him in a stroller.

My immediate thought was: he can see but I don't think he can see well. We called an eye specialist, attended the appointment, and sure enough he had vision problems. And so, at the tender age of one year and a half he was now wearing eye glasses. This was over 35 years ago. It was certainly not a common sight to see a child that young wearing spectacles back then.

I felt sad and worried for him. He would have difficulty enough keeping up physically with the other children, and now he was wearing glasses. I was concerned he would be a target for teasing until one day when he was three and a half years old.

It all started when we were at our local children's park. A gaggle of little ones and their parents, including my son and me, were enjoying a sunny afternoon at the children's park.

Children amaze me. I didn't hear it but some child must have said, "let's go to the swings." Like a flock of birds or a school of fish, the whole gaggle of little folk moved in one swift and choreographed motion toward the swings. My son tried to pivot around, his hips locked and down he went. Whap, face down into the wet sand.

Everything inside me screamed and urged me to run to him, to pick him up and dust the sand off him. I did not, I had learned he had to do these things for himself. Looking at him, I felt sad and helpless.

After his initial shock he began to lift his head. His glasses were encrusted with sand. I think it was at this point that my eyes were tearing up, and I struggled to hold back the tears.

He pulled himself up to his knees, then to his feet. He reached up, removed his glasses and rubbed the sand away from his face. It was at this moment that he looked at me.

He set his jaw, and put his glasses back on his face with intent. Then he balled up his fists on his hips and looked me straight in the eyes. I noticed it was a stern look of determination.

He lifted his left hand from his hip and pointed his finger directly at me and shouted, *"Don't you cry for me!"* And, then with further emphasis he repeated, "DON'T. YOU. CRY. FOR. ME!"

I was dumbfounded. Then I heard a high-pitched voice from the direction of the swings. His little friend Stevie was holding a swing and calling, "Come on Richard, I saved you a swing. I'll push ya. Come on."

My son cracked a broad smile and looked at me with laughing eyes. He then carefully turned and ran as best as he could to Stevie and the swing. He scrambled up onto the swing seat.

His friend pushed him and they chatted away, giggling and laughing, having a wonderful time.

WOW, I thought, what the heck just happened here? A great life lesson is what had happened, and it was a courageous and wise child who had delivered it.

I learned many things that day from the wisdom of the little fella. And I have carried these with me throughout my life.

From that day forward, I knew that my son is not bound by his physical and social challenges. He is a strong and determined person just getting on with life and with the cards life has dealt him. It is a great relief to know that throughout a lifetime there will be people and circumstances, as life will have it, that will care about him on his journey. What he needs is support in every way I can provide, and not pity. It's time to remember that these understandings apply not only to him, but to everyone, including me.

1.5 Hello Reality

With my son's wisdom in mind as I walk on the treadmill at physiotherapy, my focus wanders back to the current fact, that I just can't find a pair of shoes that feel comfortable. I guess it'll take me a while yet to not feel bound by my physical challenges. I'm working on being stronger and determined to just get on with life, with the cards life is dealing me right now. Moving on and smiling again takes a lot of hard work.

The reality at this moment is: the skin on my heels and feet are drying up and peeling away. Layer upon layer of skin is disappearing. As I take my steps forward through recovery, I need to be strong enough to walk my life forward, so it's off for an appointment with the skin specialist.

Within a couple of minutes after arriving in her office, she diagnosed me with medication-induced psoriasis. I had been on so many medications during my illness before Percy was created, and then on copious amounts after he was created.

"Jo-Ann, it's the perfect storm," she said. "There is no cure. Our course of action will be to manage it."

"So what are we going to do about this?" I asked.

"I have three separate prescriptions and a set of instructions. Three nights a week, apply this ointment, and on two nights per week, apply this other ointment. On the weekend nights, apply this third one. Wear white cotton socks during the night to keep the ointment and skin on your feet moist."

All right, one down and onto the next as I arrive at the urologist to find out why I'm not able to void properly.

"We're booking you for urology testing and procedures at the hospital. You'll get a call from my assistant within the week,"he said.

"Yes, sure, I'll go home and wait for the phone to ring," I said as I and my droopy shoulders lifted me out of the chair. I shuffled out of his office.

Ring ... Ring ... (for the umpteenth time). Now that's it, I'm not running for the phone anymore! It can just ring till I get there. Geez, it's been two weeks I've been waiting for doctors' assistants to call. It's a lot of hurry up and wait. Wait is not something I've mastered. More lessons I guess I'm destined to learn: everything in its time, patience is a virtue, and a stubbed toe really hurts after you've bumped into the door frame as you run for the phone at as full speed as is possible for me.

"Yes, I can be at the hospital for 8:30 a.m. Yes, I can do those preparations. Yes, I know the cross-city traffic is unpredictable at that time of day. Yes, we'll give ourselves an extra hour of travel time. No, we won't arrive late for the procedure. I'll set an alarm just to make sure. Thank you," I said to the lady on the other end of the phone, with squared shoulders.

We did arrive for the urology procedures about an hour early. It seemed the morning traffic was lighter than usual, go figure, I have no idea why. We had brought books and were able to get through a lot of chapters of uninterrupted reading till they called me in.

A few weeks later I was back at the urology specialists office. "We've got all of the results back, Jo-Ann. It seems the nerves that control the urinary function are not fully functional." He said this with my file open in front of him on his desk.

"Oh really. Well what do I do about this?"

"I'm hoping they will in essence wake up and kick in again. The damage from the initial disease, plus the surgery, has caused the nerve damage."

"It seems that's a recurring theme for me these days," I said with resignation.

"I'm writing a prescription for catheterization equipment. You will self-catheterize twice a day for a year. This is necessary to ensure your bladder is fully emptied. I will arrange for a home-care professional to train you how to do this. When you leave, make an appointment at the front desk and I'll see you in a year."

Oh great I thought, I poop in a bag and I pee through a plastic tube. Does it get any better than this!

Argh …

I've been through so much already, and things are getting more and more complicated. What happened to my transformation through a spectacular recovery?

1.6 Lifting my Head High

When a stoma is created, a part of an intra-abdominal structure — such as the small intestine in the case of an ileostomy and the colon in the case of a colostomy — means the intestine is intentionally brought through the abdominal wall muscles so that it can be accessible at the skin level. Percy and I call it our *outdoor plumbing*. In lay terms, the abdominal wall (including the abdominal muscle) has been compromised. It's not like a cut that can then close up, heal, and once again the abdomen is holding strong. Think of the abdominal wall as a balloon, for example, in which a hole has been made. No matter how well you patch the balloon, the integrity of the balloon skin will never be the same, it will always be weak. A hernia is a weakness in the wall of the abdomen that allows the contents to bulge out forming a lump or swelling. If the weakness occurs where the stoma is attached to the muscle wall, it will cause a swelling around the stoma, and this is called a parastomal hernia. In the case of a parastomal hernia, statistics tell us 20 to 50% of ostomates will develop a parastomal hernia. Some medical practitioners state eventually 100% of ostomates will develop a parastomal hernia.

Parastomal hernias are usually uncomfortable and can become extremely inconvenient. They may make it difficult to attach ostomy equipment and bags properly, and sometimes their sheer size is an embarrassment as they can be seen beneath clothes. Although a rare complication, the intestine can sometimes become trapped or kinked within the hernia and this in turn causes the intestine to become obstructed and to lose its blood supply (strangulated hernia), which is a dangerous and life-threatening complication.

Of course, with a parastomal hernia, trying to fit ostomy equipment that will stay fixed and hold, avoiding breaches, is a daily frustration. Every body is different, and all of the companies I have dealt with who develop and sell the ostomy products are aware of this and so produce a wide range of superior products. The companies provide phone lines whereby an ostomate can speak with the company's in-house enterostomal specialist who will ask for particulars including stoma measurements. The company will then send free sample ostomy products to the ostomate for their trial use. The in-house nurse will then follow up with a phone call within a couple of weeks. It is at this time the ostomate will know if the particular product is working for them or not. This is so very helpful for ostomates but to find equipment that works remains an individual thing. My problem is, I still haven't found equipment that works for me. Yet. With a lot of experimentation of various designs, there will be success eventually, but it will take time and potentially a few more accidents. There are many new ostomates who are as worried about a breach as I am. Some folks remain shut-in's, which is unnecessary and horrible for them. Some go out only seldom. Until we find the right equipment, for many of us, as soon as we go out the door, we worry and are anxious we'll have a breach in a public situation, and at any time. Even with the best-fitting equipment, there's always a concern of a potential accident and so, there's always a degree of anxiety an ostomate must manage. In reality, with properly fitting equipment, this is NOT a common occurrence.

My equipment issues right now are due to my lopsided contours, but there are many other reasons why equipment may not fit and the result is leakage. (For information on ostomy equipment and potential leakage, go to the "Information, Tips & Hints" section.)

I'm bothered with worrying that my parastomal hernia is growing so, every day, I monitor Percy and me for possible hernia/bowel strangulation. And, I'm concerned with having a breach, and then leakage, when I'm out and about.

Jo-Ann, we love getting out, enjoying friends, family and frankly it's about getting on with life. My job for you is to sustain your life, your job is to live it to the fullest. Come on, Jo-Ann, get on board, everything will work out. It's just going to take some time, work, and maybe a few embarrassing moments.

Thanks for that, Percy. A good reminder that this is my opportunity to give and receive the best I can, to and from life. Whether we are ostomates or not, every day when we wake up, we have another chance at participating fully in our lives, in spite of it all.

Lumpy abdomen, anxiety that at any inconvenient moment poop may occur, fear that Percy could be strangled at any time, my peeling feet, voiding through a plastic tube and my dropping foot mean I pay conscious attention to every step I take. I'm required to pick up my right foot and then my left foot. I must do this to avoid dragging my left foot, which could end up with me stumbling and tumbling. Ha, when I think about this, what an amazing metaphor for my life. As I am required to be conscious of my physical steps to get me from where I am to where I want to go, I am also conscious of my psychological steps to get me from where I am to where I want to go. Wow. Life is so fascinating.

Lifting my head high, it is time to buck up. There is a time in all of our lives when something important to us is lost. Then, there is the time when we really and truly notice the loss. We enter into upset, denial, we can even feel anger, and we grieve our loss. We experience the difficult moments when we remember what we lost, and we want to go back to the time before our loss for a visit. We strive to make peace with what has happened. Then we explore what we can do about it all so we can come out to the other side.

Who am I now? Well I'm the same Jo-Ann basically. I still have my likes and dislikes. I'm short. I'm a life partner, parent and grandparent. I am sister, daughter, neighbour and friend. I'm writer/author, artist, photographer and life coach. Gosh, I'm still who I am even though I have physical challenges now, a shock and grief to work through, and a new normal to create. I'm still me, and Percy and I simply need to make it up as we go along.

Oh, I'm so pleased you included me in your "me" thoughts, Jo-Ann. You know, many people sport their ostomies in respectful silence. Let's face it, most people really don't like us talking about it — too much information they say as they cut us off in mid-sentence. Some ostomates are worried and embarrassed. Others are concerned about their parastomal hernia bumps protruding out there for all the world to see. Let's face it, if you could have it any other way, you'd really rather not have an ostomy. But the fact remains this is part of who you are now, Jo-Ann, and what I am.

Yes, I am what I am, Percy. Some of my parts are gone, a new part was created. I'm an ostomate and I have a whole new second life to live.

1.7 Time Out!

Sitting in my backyard listening to the birds and watching the bugs buzz by, I've been flipping my eyes inward to my internal universe for the past couple of days. I've given myself a *time out* to search my mind, soul and body. I'm waiting for the light in my heart and head to turn on.

"Niki, would you like a treat?" I asked my little cat.

"Here you are, honey, don't eat it too fast. Oh yes, I love you, too." I said as she rubbed her head on my leg in gratitude.

Ah ha, that's the ticket! Every time in my life when I stop to feel and express gratitude, this feeling and act has always had a way of bringing me back home to myself. That's what I need to do, it is time once again to take stock of all the wonders of me, those who share my life, and my life in its parts and entirety. I will create a particular act of gratitude to solidify it, I will make actual and real my true feelings of gratitude. Just like my Granny taught me, "a person of words and not of deeds, is like a garden full of weeds." This will be my launch pad to get on with getting on, in spite of it all, and come what may.

I'm thinking long and hard during my time out and by the way, I'm still not rushing to the phone. The answering service can take care of that. When I'm ready I'll emerge.

I am grateful for so many things, people and events, but what stands out in my mind at this moment, is my gratitude to my life partner. Mark who has been with me throughout the time of my illness. Mark was with me, waiting anxiously in what was almost the last hour of my life. It was Mark who said what could have been our last goodbye as they wheeled me into the operating theatre. It was Mark who was with me as I began my recovery, and he welcomed Percy with an open mind, heart and arms, as part of our relationship. It was Mark who stepped up to the plate and met the demands as my caregiver. Gosh, how fortunate I am, and I'm so grateful!

Mark is a songwriter/musician and a poet, and for me to take on the challenge of writing a poem especially for him would be an action that would actively and outwardly solidify my gratitude. I've always thought that feeling gratitude is one thing, but that's not enough. The declaration of gratitude makes it actual and real for me individually, and for the world.

So, I will create a poem. That is my active declaration, It's my something that will speak grateful volumes. Yes that's it! Trouble is, I'm not a poet. I've never really written a poem in my life. I don't know the first thing about how to go about writing a poem. My mind just doesn't seem to operate in rhythm and rhyme. Hmm ... I'd better do some research and try to get the hang of it, in some small measure at any rate.

I particularly like the concept and pace of the ancient Greek odes. Just got to love the Internet, it's so useful as a tool. After some study online, and many failed attempts I finally created my ode for Mark. It is an ode to all caregivers, and here it is:

Ode To My Caregiver (Jo-Ann L. Tremblay)

Eyes glazed over and lying on my back,
Through the darkness I gaze up to you;
Conspiring together to keep me on track.
The things you want to affect are mine too,
We blend our roles as the 1000 mile healing journey begins,
Terrified, filled with fear and pain,
Your humanity glowing shines through.

Fighting for my body to take control, and keeping my mind sane,
Cold and dark when we set out, as my body strength dims,

Until I think the decent into the dark will never cease,
I look up to you as our combined strength binds.
Your steady hands and feet are mine,
Through the cloud of pain I gaze up to you;
Hard at work you are, so I may dine.
With gentle smiles you tenderly help me feel rosy blue,
Your humanity glowing shines through.

Strong laden shoulders lift the burdens from me,
Each day my healing journey continues to haste;
Committed to your charge you minister to,
With patience and dedication to set healing more;
At the end of the dying day, how can I your patient but adore,
Wrapped in the warmth of your care I feel safe.
The mood is much brighter as the days pass,
With a swell of joy and admiration I gaze up to you;
So many times through the uncertainty we found ourselves thrash,
Yet, we also found our pace forward steady and true,
Your humanity glowing shines through.

Close bosom-friend of the healing journey,
Joining me in the dance, two steps forward, a slide to the side,
Then, one step backward, followed by two more forward, now let's hurry;
Always hand in hand dear caregiver we are,
As we look to the end of our journey now not so far,
Thank you, thank you, a thousand times thank you.

1.8 It's a Matter of Pride

Wow. My state of mind is somewhat back on track, now it's time to get on with creating that, *upward turn*, from the inside and out.

With the multitude of healthcare professionals who have observed and worked with the inside, outside, and most parts of my body over the past few years, sitting on my toilet, with the healthcare nurse about 30 centimetres (12 inches) from me, instructing me on self-catheterization, is not a walk in the park for me.

She's so patient and gentle. I'm in a better frame of mind so, what the heck. I'm not the first, nor the last, person she's observing and instructing. It's a matter of pride, my dear self, so suck it up, princess.

Time for my physiotherapy appointment, and I'm on the treadmill. Have to consciously lift my left foot in order to walk without tripping and falling. Drop foot seems to be particularly bad today. The damaged nerves are just not sparking with energy. It was a year ago at this time when I was in a wheelchair. Hey, at least I'm back walking on my two feet, so suck it up, princess.

My parastomal hernia is continuing to grow. Having a terrible time with the ostomy equipment. Nothing seems to be a good fit, breaches are occurring any where and at any time. Poor Percy is so high maintenance. I'll have to make an appointment with an enterostomal nurse (ET nurse). These medical professionals are the experts in wound care and ostomies. Physicians create our ostomies, ET nurses help us take care of our ostomies.

"You need a convex barrier ring. This extra piece of equipment applied under the flange will help prevent ostomy drainage from getting under the pouch seal, protecting you from a breach," the ET nurse instructed.

Oh now I need another piece of equipment in addition to the regular ostomy equipment. How many more layers do I need? I'm going to have to wear a tent to cover all of this. Well, maybe a tent is a gross exaggeration, so suck it up, princess.

The surgeon's assistant has not called me to inform me of the surgery date yet. Good, more time to build up my body, mind, emotions and spirit in preparation for the next big one.

Ah, now that's the spirit. I'm catching on. I'm working with the professionals closely, placing my confidence in their capable hands. Time now to let my roots show, time to create and insert my individuality into the mix.

Firstly, nerves have been severed, other nerves have been damaged. In order to make progress with some of my physical issues, I need to wake those nerves up some way, somehow. I need to have my body build new neurological bridges where needed. I truly believe there's a mind/body connection and come hell or high water I'm going to find a way to make those connections that will ignite and make them spark with life again.

After thinking on this, what has come to mind is visualization. And so I've begun to visualize a vibrant tree with branches reaching out far and wide. I'm visualizing growing roots of the tree, imagining them flowing and glowing with light and energy. I don't know if this will assist in the growth and awakening of my nerves, but I sure will give it a try on a daily basis. I'm working on lighting my fire. Time will tell and who knows where this mind/body connection adventure will take me.

Realistically, although I'm in recovery mode and new physical issues seem to be appearing on a regular basis, remembering dear Mémère and her wisdom, it is time for me to be productive and achieve something. We all have our individuality and what works for one person may not be the thing that works for another. For me, being productive is one of my ways of going beyond coping to arrive at thriving. I learned this from my Father's mother through her example. When she reached her hundredth year, her mind was as sharp as it had always been. But there were days when her body did not function well. These were the days when she prayed for the ill and the needy. From her own bed, she did what she could do to be productive, to achieve, to give back to life. She did for others and in doing so, did also for her own mental, emotional self, and for her human spirit. Thanks Mémère.

I want to say something, Jo-Ann.

Yes, Percy.

I'm at the end of the digestive line. The path ends with me. You're so often scared if I'm moving too fast or too slow. You tell me I'm causing you to not be on the easy track. When you attend to me, you give big sighs and blink your eyes.

Sometimes it seems as though you blink so that when you open your eyes, you wish this all didn't really happen and it will all just go away. Well, Jo-Ann, the doctors say I'm permanent. I'm here for the long haul. I'm not going away. I'm located east southeast of your belly button and I'm here to stay. I'm new to this as well, Jo-Ann. I don't understand me, either, and I'm doing my best. It's really all up to you to get us on the straight and narrow again.

Oh Percy, yes, it is up to me. I know you're going to keep on moving and I've got to get us both moving somewhere. We're not broken for good, nor are we beyond repair. It's terrible what's happened to us, and there are so many stomas and people out there going through their own tragedies. You know, Percy, it is said: "tragedy and elation are often close neighbours." For sure I'm sorry that all of this happened to me, but I'm an active spirit, maybe I can turn it around and decide it's meant to be for the sake of others. Yes, maybe for the sake of others will also be for the sake of ourselves, Percy. That's it, from tragedy we'll create elation. We'll achieve this for our own sake, and for the sake of others. We're at the point, Percy. We know we're starting again, and we know where we're starting from. I think this is a good start. And I promise you, Percy, as we go along on this journey, I will learn everything I can about ostomies, ostomates, how to cope, accept, manage, and learn how to live with you my little stoma buddy.

Time to push away all of my doubts because my hope lies in getting started. I want to break away. Time to start something. Time to sit down with myself and decide what I am starting.

PART 2

New Horizons

2.0 Taking Flight

I had a dream last night. It was amazing. I was a bird swimming on a lake. I focused on my ears to hear the haunting cry of a loon that echoed across the lake. As I glided over the surface of the water, I looked to the land and saw the tall pines wave in the wind and the soft forest floor was dappled with sunshine. The rugged beauty changed as the sun set just in time to open up the night sky that was heavy with twinkling stars. The lake reflected the silver magic of the moon across the black water. The night ended, and the sun rose once again, burning off the early morning mist that covered the surface of the water. It was at this time I began to flap my wings that then lifted me off the surface of the water, and I headed for the sky.

Thinking on this dream, I realize I can count on the sun coming up, shining and setting every day, even when there are clouds. The stars always twinkle and shine, even when it rains. The winds of change blow causing things to bend and twist, as they create ripples of highs and lows. At times, things are hidden by a veil of mist, for a while. And we all have what it takes to lift ourselves to take flight and to reach for the sky. So another bag, another day, yet, each day like no other. As the monk who carries his buckets down the mountain dips and fills them, carries them up the mountain and empties them, life is most often hard work physically, emotionally, mentally — and goodness, how it can effect our human spirits. Yet we can rise above it all with a change of mind and heart. Richard Bach author of Jonathan Livingston Seagull, writes, "whole body, from wingtip to wingtip, is nothing more than your thought itself, in a form you can see. Break the chains of your thought, and you break the chains of your body, too."

One of my personal pressure release outlets is to write, and so, during the latter part of my illness, after the emergency surgery and during my year long recovery, each day when I was up to it, I would write a few sentences on what was happening and how I felt about it. Today, I've decided I would like to go back to my writings and give them a good read, as I think it will provide me with a foundation to begin my new self, my new normal, my breakaway to my new future.

As I read each sentence and paragraph, a powerful story of loss, desperation, endurance and humour, unfolds. It's a year-

and-a-half account of what it was to be me during that time. At that time, I think only the cells of my body carried me on, and at other times I think it was my human spirit, all on its own, that carried me. As I finished reading, I realized the writings were more than a venting exercise, they were actually an individualized account, my slice-of-life version of struggle, fear, pain, joy, the love of folks who care, and the triumph of the human spirit.

I asked Mark to read my writings as I wanted to know what he thought. When he finished reading, he said, ", Jo-Ann. You've written a book."

Inside of me, that's what I feel about the writings.

We've got it, Percy. This is our launch pad! We decided our intent is to turn my adversity around so that it will be valuable to you, me, our life, and for the people who are a part of it. I think what I've written will have a good measure of value for anyone who has, is now, or is destined to face the realities of adversity whether it is chosen or thrust upon them. We have a book.

I have been a Life and Corporate Coach for private and professional clients since 1987. People are amazing to me and each person is on a remarkable journey that is their life. During their lives they develop talents, skills, abilities, individualities, and strategies. These become the tools they put into their personal and professional toolbox. As the events of their lives unfold, when they need a particular tool or tools, they reach in and pull out the one that will work for them. Unfortunately, we don't always have the right tool we need. Sometimes we don't recognize a tool we possess, and at other times, we just don't know how to apply the tool(s). And so, in 2004 I had decided to write a book titled, *The Self-Coaching Toolbox, Six tools for personal and professional growth & development*. It is a book dedicated to assisting people to personally and professionally coach themselves. It's a self-management and self-motivational book that folks can use to maximize their potential for achieving their own defined meaningful success.

As I had never pursued publishing a book before that time, I decided to become a member of the Canadian Authors Association (CAA). I needed to learn all I could about the author and book publishing field. Over time, I became a member of the Executive in my Ottawa region. As I continued my work with the Association I took on the responsibility of vice-president of podcasts for the National Capital Region branch. It was a delightful time, a pleasure and an honour to work with the Associations' members and Executive. There were so many folks at all stages of authoring, writing and publishing, who were ready and willing to take a novice such as myself under their wing and guide me. I was eventually accepted by a publisher and the book was completed and published in 2005.

Now I have another book written, and one of the first steps is to secure myself a professional editor. One of the Executive members I met at CAA and worked with on a number of projects is, Sherrill Wark, and I'm delighted and honoured to know her. Sherrill is a knowledgeable, talented, and incredibly funny person. Among many of her talents, she is a writer, published author, poet, animal lover/advocate, and an editor. One of my favourites of her many published works is, *Really Stupid Writing Mistakes: How to Avoid Them*. I think that book was truly written for people like me.

The manuscript is ready and with my trust in Sherrill and her expert editing abilities, I've decided to connect with her at her company Crowe Creations, to ask if she'd give my manuscript a read and decide if she would take me on as a client. It didn't take long — happy, happy, she's accepted, and the manuscript and the editing is a go!

Oh, Percy, here we are. As they say, if you're handed lemons, make lemonade. Well, we've been handed a boatload of lemons in the past few years.

I guess we're going to have to make a tanker full of lemonade, Jo-Ann.

Ha, you're cute, Percy.

Our work has begun. Now I fancy myself as a pretty good writer, but I must say, no matter how good one is, always, always, submit and work with a professional editor. I sometimes think I know the written English language and then when an editor such as the talented Sherrill goes over the work, well, let's just say thank goodness for editors. It's September 10, and Sherrill is now reviewing and editing the manuscript. I'm so excited that our experience and the fact that I'm alive to share it in the form of a book is happening.

We're on the good road now Percy.

Our next step is to decide on how we will publish the book. Today, writers are living in a really great time, when it comes to publishing our work. When *The Self-Coaching Toolbox* was published in 2005, self-publishing was not held in high regard by the publishing industry, or by the general public. The industry has come a long way since, thanks in part to the Internet.

It used to be, a writer sent their manuscripts to a specific publisher who specialized in the writer's genre. Then the publisher would accept a set number of manuscripts they would publish in that year. The odds of being accepted by a publishing company were and are limited. The greatest challenges for a writer is to market, print, store, and distribute his or her book. Unless the writer is a really well-known author, the odds of being financed and sent on a book signing tour by the publishing company are slim to none. Even with a publisher, most lesser-known authors were and are required to network and market themselves and their book. The publisher has contacts and is able to attend various book conferences, for example, and they will bring with them their printed catalogue of their stable of authors and their titles. This would consist of your book cover art, a short synopsis, and your bio on a page, but again, the odds of anyone really noticing your book if you're not an already established author ... Well let's just say the likelihood is remote.

The greatest asset the publisher has for the author is printing and distribution. How do our books get out to market? And how do people learn about the author and the book itself? *The Self-Coaching Toolbox*, for example, is available in bookstores such as Chapters Indigo, but as shelf space is limited, there are only so many book titles available on store shelves, as space is costly for the industry. Many available books for purchase are not on the shelves; therefore, the books must be ordered by the purchaser. If a person who may be interested in your book's subject matter doesn't know your book exists because the book is not on a shelf, they of course cannot pick up it up for a quick scan to see if they'd like to purchase it ... well there's another potential reader who's not buying and reading your book. Therefore, the odds of their finding out about you the author and your book, once again, are slim to none.

Today, we have the option for self-published printed books and e-books, otherwise known as Indie publishing. Many folks have e-book readers and are enjoying reading from them. In my case, although my paper books are my treasures, I also love my e-book reader. I have a library of over a hundred books that I carry in a little case with me, and I have access to all of them at my fingertips. Wow. Don't we live in amazing times?

And so, after careful research, I decided I would self-publish *Better WITH a Bag than IN a Bag, From the brink of death to recovery through humour and inspiration*. There was certainly a learning curve, but I must say the self-publishing industry really makes it accessible to everyone. Our choice to begin the publishing adventure was with Amazon and the book can be ordered by readers from there. We would not only have distribution in the United States and Canada, the paperback and e-book format are also available with Amazon around the world in countries such as; the United Kingdom, France, Germany, Spain, Australia, and Japan. Amazon Kindle also has a lending library. After a three-month period, the book is then available through other e-book and print book sellers, (for example Kobo, iTunes). At this juncture I'm also researching networking, marketing and publicity.

For the first time in what feels a long time, my thinking, time and energy is being placed outside and off of myself and my physical challenges. I've always felt that when I'm feeling unwell, if I redirect my attention and activities beyond myself, I can cope much better than by being fixated on me and wallowing in my problem(s).

So onwards and upwards we go, Percy.

2.1 Meanwhile

I still have not received the phone call informing me of the surgery date for the parastomal hernia repair. Must say, after going through so much before, during and after my last surgery, I'm really quite frightened about the potential what-ifs that must be considered for any surgical procedure. This wait isn't helping. I'm still catheterizing myself multiple times a day. Percy's ostomy equipment is failing more times in a week than we can count. Although I'm following the physicians psoriasis cream therapy program, the skin on my heels, feet and on the palms of my hands continue to peel off layer by layer. Skin is composed of three primary layers, I think I have only one layer left in those areas. One nick by a toe nail and my skin tears open, and healing seems to take forever. With each physiotherapy session, I can feel my body getting stronger, preparing me for the major surgical adventure that lies ahead of me. I continue to envision vibrant branches and roots of a tree as part of my personal contribution to nerve damage healing, which at this time doesn't seem to be getting me anywhere. I am having to be ever so conscious of lifting my feet in order to stave off the horror of tripping over my drop foot and injuring Percy and me. To add to our difficulties, my bowel movements are completely inconsistent. Sometimes loose, sometimes hard, and other times no movement at all. Unfortunately, it's now off to the gastroenterologist at the Ottawa Hospital to try to figure things out.

Percy and I are determined not to be discouraged from the roll we're on so I applied and was accepted to place an oil painting I had painted in the year during my initial recovery period, to be part of a juried awards exhibition with the Arteast group of artists I am a member of. The name of the piece is "Window on the World". At this time in my life, this is a most appropriate subject matter and name for my piece of art. In fact, as I think about the cover art for *Better WITH a Bag than IN a Bag*, when the manuscript is ready for publication, I'm considering putting a particular piece of art I also painted during the first year of my recovery process.

Oh, oh, me, me, pick me, Jo-Ann.

Pick you for what, Percy?

I would like to share our art story since I'm going to be the star of the book cover.

Well yes, Percy. You are the star of the book cover. Sure you can share our artistic endeavours that occurred during the first year of our recovery.

As Jo-Ann mentioned, redirecting her mind, going into action and being productive is part of a formula that works well for taking her mind off herself when times are tough. As she continued to recuperate from her illness and surgery, she had many night dreams. I think the dreams had a lot to do with the medications she was required to take. At any rate, there was a particular dream in which she splished and splashed through a kaleidoscope landscape of thick and colourful semi-liquid substances. At one point in the dream, she looked to her right and there, glistening in the sunlight, was a set of knives. Now the knives were not aggressive in nature. They were simply shiny tools beside her. When she awoke, she could not shake the dream from her mind. As she thought deeply on it, she decided the details meant something to her. She had only to figure it out. Possibly her subconscious was trying to relay a message, or messages, to her. Jo-Ann believes dreams provide people with information symbolically, and so she decided her inner self was trying to tell her something or some things.

Within a few days of thinking about the recurring dream, she realized the colourful and somewhat mucky substance throughout the dreamscape was all about texture. Well, Jo-Ann knows I'm all about texture, and right out there in front of her. The knives were quite easy to decipher. Surgical knives had been used to save her life and they had altered her physiology. With the expert hands of a surgeon, they had carved Jo-Ann into a survivor. Armed with these understandings, Jo-Ann realized, as part of her recovery, she would now take up oil painting with palette knives, a new medium and art tool adventure for her.

She had been a watercolour artist for a number of years. She now decided, through the messages of her dreams, it was time to change the thin consistency of watercolour paint as a medium to the thick consistency of oil paints, the consistency that very closely resembles the dreamscape she sploshed through in her dream. She pondered what her first painting would be and then it dawned on her, I'm her inspiration — and as they say, when an individual starts any new venture, one should start with what they know — Jo-Ann decided on painting me and eventually the piece of art became what we call, "Percy, A Self-Portrait". Yes, she painted me!

Jo-Ann was in recovery, and she found painting me was important to her and it eventually bloomed into a cathartic experience, and it still is. Healing became both fun and productive, in spite of the hardships, at that time. Being able to paint and being productive was, and is, wonderful. Splishing, sploshing and splashing through the thick rainbow of colours using knives has been very valuable and therapeutic for her emotionally, so physically as well.

She has continued to paint with oil and knives, and eventually she decided her next set of art pieces would have the theme of doors and windows. Let's face it, a door (so to speak) was closed when part of her colon was amputated, and a window in the form of me became her colostomy opening.

With me as her inspiration, she chose to create a series of four separate symbolic paintings. Each one of these pictures features masonry walls with doors and windows. Masonry walls are symbolic of the abdominal wall, and windows and doors represents the various entrances and exits of the human internal universe. "Window on the World" is one of those pictures from the series that is now hanging on the gallery wall alongside the artistic creations of her artist compatriots. It is being judged by art experts and viewed by our community of humanity. It is exciting for us to risk ourselves and put new, never before tried by Jo-Ann, out there for all to experience.

Thank you, Percy, for sharing. Yes, I'm inspired by "Percy A Self-Portrait" and I'm so pleased to include it as the artwork on the cover of the book. One would think a stoma and equipment is not very easy on the eyes. Let's face it, Percy, you're not considered the most handsome.

Gee, thanks, Jo-Ann.

Sorry, Percy, but I hadn't finished yet.

Proceed.

A stoma is often referred to as a "rosebud" as it is a close imagery depiction of what a stoma itself looks like, in reality a not so beautiful rosebud, but rosebud-ish.

Hey!

As I was saying, a stoma is referred to as a "rosebud", and when the reader looks at the book cover right side up, they will see a stoma. When they turn the book upside down, what was Percy in a downward direction, which is how my Percy is seated, you now see a beautiful red rose bud. For me, it's a wonderful metaphor for the reality of having a colostomy and living my life as an ostomate. What I mean by this is: I am an ostomate now and for the rest of my life, and what comes with this is the daily challenges an ostomy imposes, and the stigma that can be a part of this. Conversely, the rosebud symbolizes the blessed joy of being alive, that we have a second chance to live and experience life in spite of it all. (For more information about stigma, go to the "Information, Tips & Hints" section.)

Jo-Ann.

Yes, Percy.

Can I, your little rosebud, share a little about what we learned about red roses with everyone?

Sure, Percy.

It's said that the red rose not only carries more meaning than any other colour of rose, it is also one of the most universal of all symbols. First, the red rose has provided a wealth of significance as it is and has been represented in countless works of art from classical paintings and poetry to modern day music and media. In fact, the Ostomy Canada Society (OCS) displays a red rose in the middle of a bouquet of white roses on their website http://www.ostomycanada.ca and in their brochure with the caption: "Do you feel like the only one?" The Ostomy Canada Society (OCS) welcomes everyone and is there to help and support ostomates, their families, caregivers and friends.

Red roses have appeared throughout history and across many cultures as political and religious symbols. The mystique of the red rose *(oh, I like the sound of that)* has been a source of immeasurable inspiration for many throughout the ages. However, it is as the symbol of love that the red rose is most commonly recognized. In Greek and Roman mythology, the red rose was closely tied to the goddess of love. This thinking and these feelings have endured to the present day. Red roses continue to be the most popular way to say "I love you" to someone special. So, Jo-Ann, when you think of me, when you attend to me, I'm always telling you "I love you."

Oh, Percy, that's so sweet, thank you.

As Percy and I continue to move ahead on our book project, it's time to design the back cover of the book. I've been thinking and I'd really like to ask two individuals who have experience and an intimate knowledge of what an ostomy is, two who know what it's like to be an ostomate. I'd like them to read the manuscript, review it, then provide their comments for the back cover. In addition, since I have a sense of humour when it comes to life's ups and downs, I think I'd like to ask a third person, one who's been on a tough life journey himself, one who can make lemonade out of lemons through being tough and inspirationally humorous. Aha, I know the folks I'd like to approach.

One of the individuals I know who is knowledgeable about ostomies and ostomates is Andrea Manson. I've had the honour and pleasure of speaking with and doing some business with Andrea. She is an enterostomal therapy nurse living and conducting her business Care and Supply Centre in New Westminster, British Columbia, Canada. Andrea has been instrumental in helping me acquire an appropriate ostomy hernia support belt. It is recommended that ostomates not lift anything too heavy without wearing a support belt and at the time I connected with her, I was starting to develop my doozy of a parastomal hernia, so I sure needed to wear one for support. Finding the support that works for me took quite a bit of research, and through the research I was able to connect with Andrea and her ostomy care and supply company. Once again, thank you to the Internet. With passion and compassion, Andrea is committed to people and their lifelong ostomy journey. She is extremely knowledgeable, very connected to the ostomy community, and is patient and helpful. She was precious to me when I was lost in the ostomy support jungle and has continued to stay connected with me. So I've decided, when Sherrill and I are finished editing the manuscript, I'll give Andrea a shout and ask her if she'll read the manuscript and provide the project with her back cover comments/review.

It's also an honour to know Mike MacDonald, one of Canada's premier comedians. He's hailed in some quarters as the "King of Canadian Comedy". He has performed all over North America as well as appearing on the *Late Show With David Letterman, The Arsenio Hall Show, A&E's An Evening at the Improv,* and multiple *Comedy Central* television specials. He has hosted both the *Canadian Gemini Awards* and the *Just For Laughs 10th Anniversary Special for CBC,* and has done so much more ... Life has not always been easy for him, and things went seriously downhill for Mike a few years ago when he collapsed onstage one day. He had liver poisoning. His liver subsequently became infected, then his kidneys shut down. He has Hepatitis C, he needed and received a liver transplant. The Canadian Liver Foundation (CLF) and Canadian comedian Mike MacDonald are calling upon everyone to learn more and get tested for Hepatitis C, a potentially fatal liver disease. The organization has launched an awareness campaign which includes a Canadian national public service announcement (PSA) featuring the comedian (http://www.liver.ca). Mike has always provided me with the most potent medicine of all: humour.

I of course by now have met fellow ostomates. One of them is Carol A Stephen, a Canadian Authors Association member who is an award winning poet. *Above the Hum of Yellow Jackets,* published by Bondi Studios, and *Architectural Variations,* Quillfire Publishing, are just a couple of her published books. In addition, some of her poems are on-line at *The Light Ekphrastic.* She has and continues to be involved with poetry and poetry books. Carol is a member of the League of Canadian Poets and was a featured reader as one of Reading Series' *Hot Ottawa Voices.* Carol has been an ostomate for many years now; she sure knows the challenges, and as a writer and poet, I really feel she's knowledgeable and will shoot straight from the hip as a commentator and reviewer of the manuscript.

All right, we're still on track here, Percy.

Hey, I'm glad to hear it, Jo-Ann. In fact, I'm hearing a bit of a lilt to your voice.

Yes, Percy, in spite of our ongoing issues, I feel grateful. Through our intent on finding all of the ways possible for us to share and, of course, the distraction from my "self" concerns, I do know that although in some ways nothing has really changed, I also know that in all ways everything is changing.

The ever efficient Sherrill has completed the editing of *Better WITH a Bag than IN a Bag* and I've sent the manuscripts to Andrea, Mike and Carol. It's a really big job that takes up their precious time and knowledge to commit to reading a manuscript and to review and comment on it. I am forever grateful to Andrea Manson, Mike MacDonald and Carol A Stephen for their interest and support with their wonderful contribution to our ostomy awareness and advocacy book project. We're hitting the ground running, drop foot and all, and it feels good.

2.2 The Learning Curve

Percy and I continue our ostomy learning and marketing strategy. I'm on social media, my Facebook page is "Author Jo-Ann L Tremblay", and I've begun to seek out the potential for ostomy and bowel disease Facebook groups. Well, I sure hit the jackpot. There are many active groups. (For a list of the groups I have found, go to "Information, Tips & Hints" section.)

These ostomy and bowel disease groups are designed to be a community support group run for the benefit of ostomates and sufferers of various bowel diseases, their caregivers, families and friends. The administrators of these groups promote respect for each other's feelings and ask people to think before they post. The groups are made up of people from around the world and are created for people with stomas (colostomy, ileostomy, urostomy) and/or folks with bowel diseases, and are dedicated to sharing thoughts, ideas, tips, challenges, ostomy fashion and inspiration for being fit and active.

Participants may discuss foods, health issues, lifestyle, emotions, seek support, and more. Of course, the administrators of the groups recommend that for a medical opinion, a person speak to their enterostomal nurse, doctor, or appropriate medical professional.

I've made friends with folks from all parts of the world as a member of the various Facebook groups. We talk, share, exchange ideas and support one another.

Next, my research brought me to Twitter. Inc., this is an online social networking service that enables users to send and receive short 140-character messages called "tweets". Registered users can read and post tweets. Unregistered users can only read them.

I found a treasure trove of ostomates active on Twitter Inc. Situated all over the world, I've made friends with them as well. They keep me informed on what's happening in the ostomy world where they live and we share thoughts and interesting tidbits. My twitter address is @joanntremblay.

Of course, I researched books on the subject of ostomy. In addition, I used the Internet as a tool and encountered various ostomy and bowel disease forums. There is a lot of information so a person really has to take time to sift through it all and use common sense when it comes to some of the information. Through my web search, I came upon various websites dedicated to ostomies and ostomates and I found four very interesting, informative, and well-organized sites: one in Canada, one in the United States and two in the United Kingdom. All of these websites offer comprehensive information on stoma lifestyle issues.

Internet-based support websites for ostomates of all types:

• A Guide To Living With A Stoma, http://www.living-with-a-stoma.co.uk and the sister website, A Guide To Living With A Stoma, More For You, http://www.livingwithastoma.co.uk

• Ostomy Canada Society Inc. (and in French it is La Société Canadienne des Personnes Stomisées) http://www.ostomycanada.ca

• United Ostomy Association of America (UOAA), http://www.ostomy.org

(For more information and a list of websites, go to "Information, Tips & Hints" section.)

2.3 Blog, Blogger, Blogueur

Hey, Jo-Ann, what does blogueur mean?

Well, it's actually the French translation for blogger. I thought I'd be cute with this title and write out the word "blogger" in various languages. Blogs are usually a discussion or informational site published on the World Wide Web and available for people around the world to read and enjoy, so I thought I'd write the word out in various languages. Well, it really didn't work out as I've found out that many languages use the word "blog" and "blogger" and don't worry about translating it.

Well, Blog, Blogger, Blogueur has a nice ring to it, at any rate, Jo-Ann. So why are we writing here about blogs and bloggers?

I've decided we're taking flight as high as we can to create our new normal, to well ... to take our lemons to make lemonade as we go along. I feel in addition to our learning as much as we possibly can about ostomy and ostomates, and as we commit to being active with awareness and advocacy, I've decided it is time to think about creating a blog. I do feel a blog will give us an additional platform for our awareness and advocacy efforts. It will be a valuable communication tool with folks we normally would not have the opportunity to reach. A blog will help us share so much with people. As well, it's a way for people from around the world to learn about us, Percy, and the book.

Hey, that sounds great. Can I be part of it, too?

"I've been thinking about you, Percy, and how you can fit in and be active with what I'm doing. I would like to give you a public voice. I feel there is great value in your being able to speak stoma to stoma, as well as, stoma to ostomate. You can share in a way that is very valuable to ostomates. You're an experienced stoma on the move, to be sure. Actually, based on your experience, I think we'll give you the well-earned title, Percy Stoma, EoL Poopology, EoL stands for Experience of Life.

Wow, I like that!

I've started the research and there are many blog development and publishing sites available. Percy and I have decided on, Wordpress. Wordpress was first released on May 27, 2003 by its founders Matt Mulenweg and Mike Little. It is a free and open source blogging tool and a content management system (CMS). Its features include a plugin architecture and a template system. Which for me, who is quite non-technical, means it's easy to navigate and set up.

The more I think about the blog, I feel I'd like to title it, *The Ostomy Factor*. Factor meaning: a circumstance, fact, or influence that contributes to a result or outcome. "Factor" fits well with how I feel about my ostomy, and how I am required to live now.

I've never been a blogger. There's a lot to think about and learn before I start. When writers decide on a writing project, they must set a goal as to their intent for the article, blog, book, etc. They will then choose a core message for the piece. Writers must say what they want, mean what they say, but it's all in how they deliver the message. A writer will also have her own personality, her way of looking at things, and her writing style. When it comes to a blog, I'm learning that there are logistical designs to incorporate into the blog site, and so on.

Percy, I just realized it's been 15 months since you were created.

Yes, Jo-Ann, time marches on and so are we. By the way, I heard that Sherrill, our editor, has now fully completed working with the manuscript. We're ready to go! Just a little more research with regard to self-publishing and we'll be ready to publish Better WITH a Bag than IN a Bag: From the Brink of Death to Recovery Through Humour and Inspiration. Our target is November 2012. Whoopie that's in just one month. We're continuing on our way.

2.4 November 2012, A Banner Month

Jo-Ann.

Yes, Percy.

I'm so pleased you're including me in The Ostomy Factor *blog, I remember a time not so long ago where you didn't even want to look at me.*

Yes, just over a year ago, when I was post surgery and within days of Percy's creation, I was on a roller coaster of emotional intensity, I didn't know what was up or down. I felt I had to take it one step at a time. It wasn't a time to rush things. Frankly, my stoma wasn't going anywhere! The stark reality of today is, and for the rest of my life: my stoma is here to stay and if it weren't for Percy, I wouldn't be here, either. There was such a powerful shadow over me, and then there were the many adjustments I had to contend with. I eventually talked myself into taking on an attitude and repeated to myself, *I'm in charge here.* I did know that my confidence would come back to me in time and with practise, which would eventually make the adjustments easier. I remember the first time I changed my ostomy bag. I must say I gagged. I felt dirty and smelly. This was a really big step for me as it was so scary. I remember repeating to myself: I can do it and I'll get better each time. There's always the firsts for everything in life, and every time I feel sad, I'll just remember that the little stoma with its bag saved my life. I can get through this, I'll take baby steps. Let's face it, even baby steps will get me somewhere.

Over time, changing Percy's equipment has become a walk in the park. It's just part of getting dressed and then I'm ready to face the world. I'm lopsided with my ever-growing parastomal hernia; my left foot more often than not drags; and yet, I'm feeling free, happy and ready to live!

Jo-Ann, I noticed you were humming a little tune earlier when you changed my bag. That's the spirit.

Oh, you noticed, Percy.

It's November 2012! A big month for Percy and me. We've published *Better WITH a Bag than IN a Bag: From the Brink of Death to Recovery Through Humour and Inspiration* in Kindle format and in paperback format with Amazon. At the time of writing this book, *Another Bag, Another Day*, the books are also available through Kobo, iTunes, Barnes and Noble, Half.com, Alibris.com and Alibris UK.

We're moving forward on our journey through ostomy awareness and advocacy. This is so exciting and gratifying for us. Our commitment is coming alive. The new normal has begun and we're turning lemons into lemonade.

November 2012 continues to be a banner month, as we've now published our first *The Ostomy Factor* post, titled "Chances Are". The following is my first ever blog, enjoy.

Chances Are
My name is Jo-Ann L. Tremblay, I am an ostomate, and my stoma's name is "Percy", Percy's name origin/meaning — Old English derived from latin, "Persius", meaning; "to penetrate/ pierce the hedge".

My colostomy was created during life saving surgery July 21, 2011. It has been just over a year and my recovery is well on its way. It's time for celebrating life. It's my second chance, the bonus, the icing on the cake, the cherry on top. My first chance was amazing, my second chance incredible. Life is fragile, limited and precious. Always have had the time of my life, why not, it's the only life I thought I had. Now, with a second chance I'm having the time of my life, why not, it's the only life I know I have.

We get only one life to live, yet, every day we wake up with another chance to give and receive the best we can to and from life. They say, "In the end, we only regret the chances we didn't take". Those of us who have an ostomy know what another chance is. We know we've been given another opportunity to laugh and play. We know we have another chance to suffer and cry. We know we have another crack at living and then dying. Through our rebirth we have been given the experiential mileage required to make the informed decisions necessary to make the best of life that we possibly can. "Chances Are", is our credo. How phenomenal is this? How gifted we are! As I look back on the journey that brought us to the creation of our ostomies, how awful and incredible it was. At times we want to forget all of it, it has left bad stuff in our mind. The journey was jaw-dropping, amazing, and horrible.

Percy and I have created this blog, The Ostomy Factor, for the purpose of sharing with our fellow ostomates. We have had many adventures and misadventures, as so many ostomates can relate to. Our aim is to connect with ostomates, their caregivers, the medical community, and with anyone who has endured loss or major changes in their lives, and from time to time we'll talk stoma to stoma. Sharing with the stomas of the world is Percy's contribution. He has a sense of humour and is quite the little pooper. He's also very clever holding an EoL in Poopology, (EoL. Experience Of Life).

Our mission is to share the ostomate's life, times, ups, downs, and all arounds with the ostomy community through humour and inspiration.

Jo-Ann L Tremblay

Ostomate
"Everyone You Meet Has A Story To Tell"

I decided to sign off each of my posts reminding everyone who reads them that everyone has a story. I've been very fortunate in my life as I have had the honour of travelling extensively on planet Earth. Many of the travels were for pleasure and many were business trips. I've lived, played and worked with people of various religions, cultures, political leanings, and in many climates. Every single person I've met has had to face and endure something(s) that have demanded their resourcefulness and courage. A number of years ago, I produced and hosted a radio program, *Voices Of Our Town*, on a news-talk radio station in Ottawa, Canada. I had the privilege of meeting and interviewing people from 2 to 102 years of age, and each and every one of them had an amazing life experience/story to share. I believe we all have a life and a life around us. All of the people I've met have had a story to tell, and they have touched my heart and fed my soul.

2.5 The Banner Month Continues

The youngest daughter of our blended family, Meredith Henderson and her husband James Henderson, surprised me with a "book trailer" video featuring *Better WITH a Bag than IN a Bag.* [A book trailer is a video book promotion that employs techniques similar to those of movie trailers.] Book trailers can be utilized in many ways including as a YouTube video. Meredith and James operate Sisbro & Co., Inc., a production company operating out of Los Angeles, California,

USA. You can view the video on YouTube, or you can also view the video on *The Ostomy Factor* blog site. Simply click on the photo of me at the top right hand side of the "Home" page and you'll be linked with YouTube. Enjoy.

A picture is worth a thousand words historically, presently, and I'm pretty sure for the foreseeable future. As I'm learning, these days people in general are embracing visual content and according to my research, having a video and posting it, provides a valuable platform for informing people of your products and services.

Meredith took on the challenge of creating the book trailer titled, The story unfolds ... http://youtu.be/gwrW4Xmfne4. Clever and creative, Meredith put the song "Last Words", performed by my favourite band Tangleroot (music and lyrics by Noah Henderson, lead vocals Beth Henderson), to the visuals and the video story unfolds of that fateful day when I teetered on the brink of death, when my life was saved, and when my little pooper, Percy Stoma, was created.

As the month progressed, I was contacted by Mr. Ian Settlemire, editor of *Phoenix* magazine, who had read the first blog post. Phoenix magazine is the official publication of the United Ostomy Association of America (UOAA). This well-designed and informative ostomy magazine covers many ostomy-related topics from personal stories of recovery, to diet and exercise, to skin-care treatment, and more. The magazine is published quarterly — March, June, September and December. The editor read *Better WITH a Bag than IN a Bag* and published a lovely review of the book. Percy and I are new to the ostomy scene and we are very grateful for all of the support and encouragement.

A few days later, I was contacted by Mr. Qais Ghanem, author of five books to date and at the time a program host for CHIN Radio, Ottawa. . Qais's program is *Dialogue with Diversity*. He asked me to join him on his radio show to be interviewed about being an ostomate and ostomies. I was quite excited and oh so nervous! This was the first time I would be talking to a large audience and sharing myself as an ostomate.

I think I got quite excited, too, Jo-Ann.

Yes, Percy, you certainly did! Oh well, after a few rushed moments just before air time, we dealt with it in the radio station washroom. I guess I can say, with your little escapade, Percy, you helped put me in the ostomy sharing mode, with a few laughs to add to the experience.

With November almost a memory, each day is filled and Christmas is on the way.

Percy, our time for celebration, good food, family and friends is just about upon us. It's the second Christmas at our second chance at life. We're celebrating and life is good.

Let the good times roll, Jo-Ann.

2.6 One Bag, Two Bags, Three Bags Full

It's December and I still have not received the phone call informing me of the date for the parastomal hernia repair/ abdominal and stoma support surgery. I continue to feel anxiety about the potential upcoming surgery, the what-ifs and the potential for things going wrong due to hernia complications that could occur before the surgery can be performed. The hurry up and wait just isn't helping me. I'm still catheterizing multiple times a day. Percy's ostomy equipment continues to fail often due to my changing abdominal profile, and with the Christmas holidays coming up, the worry that I may have a public ostomy equipment failure while shopping or at a Christmas party, is really nipping at my heels.

Although I'm following the physician's psoriasis cream therapy program, the skin on my heels, feet, and on the palms of my hands continue to peel off layer by layer. I'm continuing with my pre-op physiotherapy sessions and this is really paying off as my body is getting stronger by the week. I'm also working hard on my vibrant branches and roots of a tree visualization in support of my body's nerve regrowth and repair. With drop foot, well I guess my Christmas dance card won't be filled this year but I can still do some sit-down swaying with some wild and abandoned toe tapping to the music thrown in for good fun.

I've met with the gastroenterologist to discuss my inconsistent bowel movements, and the outcome is really quite unsatisfying. Basically, I'm given to understand that it's all too bad but there is nothing more the medical folks can do for me. I have to take a stool softener when needed, and then a stool-hardening medication when needed and an ongoing fibre support concoction. The various ingredients of powders must be mixed together, minced, then dissolved in a liquid so I can enjoy drinking the grainy-textured assemblage every day to help my slow, sluggish, and frankly, just not working the way it should, colon. No problem. Hey! I've got this. Sheesh!

We've just gotten great news. Eldest daughter of our blended family, Beth, and her fiancé, Chris, have confirmed the wedding date. It will be celebrated next June 2013, six months from now. I'm alive and I have another joyous life experience to look forward to.

Oh my, Percy. I wonder when the surgery will be scheduled. Oh, I do hope it'll be early spring. That will give you and me time to do some healing before the big occasion.

Might be time to make another phone call, Jo-Ann.

Hmm ... We've been pinning our hopes on being able to escape the extreme cold and snow in January by heading off to warm and sunny Florida, USA, for six weeks. Eating fresh fruit and vegetables while being able to take long hikes and sunset walks on the beach will assist us to prepare for the surgery. We have a beautiful wedding to be ready for in the late spring. I need to have a date for my surgery. Okay. That's it, Percy. I'm calling the surgeon's assistant!

You go, girl. I'm right here with you. In more ways than one!

"Well hello, Jo-Ann." The surgeon's assistant said on the other end of the phone.

"Do you have any idea of when my surgery will be scheduled?" I asked.

"Oh, Jo-Ann. I know it's been a long wait. Certainly December is out, and I'm sure it won't be scheduled for January either," she said.

"We're planning to spend the month of January in Florida. I'll not be in phone contact, will you be calling me in January?"

"Jo-Ann, go to Florida and enjoy your time there. I'll be working on this end of things. In fact, I'm going to walk your file down to the surgery booking department right now. I'll give you a call in a day or two if I hear anything from them. Just go, and when you arrive back home in February, I'll probably have the surgery date and particulars ready for you then."

Goody, goody. Oh, my. I can feel my happy-toe starting to tap and it's not even Christmas yet. Hmm ... After stewing over the wait for surgery, I'm somewhat perplexed as to why I seem to be so relieved at hearing that the surgery won't happen for another few more months. The not knowing is the place that has caused me anxiety and now I feel I've regained a sense of calm. This information means I will be able to enjoy the Christmas season relatively healthy. It means we can, in fact, head off to the warmth and sunshine of the southern United States, escape the cold, snow and ice of home. It means I have more time to build my body, mind, emotions and spirit to face another round of major surgery. Life has a way of working things out in the highest and best way in spite of my insistent desire to direct it from my naive human vantage point. What will be will be and I'm going to focus on me, the me that is working so very hard to recover, the part that is getting on with my life with Percy, and to rise up and take flight to grasp a sustainable quality of life.

With each physiotherapy session under the expert direction of Sarah, I can feel my body getting stronger, preparing me for the major surgical adventure that lies ahead of me. I continue to envision vibrant branches and roots of a tree, which at this time doesn't seem to be getting me anywhere. I continue to be ever so conscious of lifting my feet.

That's it! The phone is ringing, Percy. I have a feeling I'm going to hear about the surgery. Let's get this show on the road.

"Hello? Yes. I understand. Well I must say the timing works fine for me. Thank you and Merry Christmas to you, too."

Percy, they don't have a specific date to give us yet but the surgery will happen for sure sometime early spring. When we arrive back home in February, we're to call the surgeon's office and we'll be scheduled for the pre-op appointment, and we'll be given the surgery date at that time. Wow. This is great. We have a time frame to aim for. And it's not going to interfere with Christmas plans, or our trip to Florida. Couldn't have planned it better myself. I don't feel so adrift anymore. We have a destination to navigate our way to. I can enjoy the season and use my time in Florida to prepare my whole self and you, Percy, for the surgery.

Hey. That is terrific, Jo-Ann. Christmas. That's great, too ... but I'm a little concerned about all of the rich foods you eat at that time.

Good heads up, Percy!

Christmas and New Year's is a time for family, friends, fun, and rich food. Although I must watch my food intake very carefully, digestion continues to pose a challenge for Percy and me. Inevitably, I eat something with artificial colouring, flavouring or preservatives, and these are trigger foods for me, and then it's watch out, Percy!

In fact, this is what happened December 27, a day that had promised to be filled with the children and grandchildren of my blended family. Let's start at the beginning. It was December 26 and I thought I had been very careful so Percy had been quiet. Mark, daughter Beki and daughter Meredith had performed at Maxwell's Bistro, Ottawa with Johnny Vegas and his All Star Band. Percy and I did a little dancing to the music with as many of the family as could make it out that evening.

Periodically during the evening, I visited the bathroom facilities to check on my bud, Percy. All was calm, all was right, but around yon corner ... Midnight struck, and it was time to head home. Curled up with some of the kids and Mark in the living room, fire in the fireplace, we settled in for a cozy chit chat, then off to bed we went. Tomorrow promised to be a big day. We'd be off to see Beki, her husband, Adam, and our grandchildren, Austin and Emelyn at their home for a Christmas blow out. In more ways than one, as it turned out. There, waiting to join us, were other members of the family, as more of the children and grandchildren had arrived from out of town. There would be fourteen of us at the Christmas dinner table. But as it turned out, Percy had other ideas.

No sooner had I put the fire out, turned off the lights and crawled into bed, still filled with the music of the night, when Percy went flipping berserk! I hardly slept a wink through the night, spending most of it wearing a path from the bed to the bathroom and back again. Must say my enthusiasm for the Christmas celebration the next day was slowly but surely ebbing as the night continued.

By the time morning arrived, my body, mind and poor little Percy were a dragged-out mess. I had no choice. I stayed in my pyjamas as I waved good bye to Mark, Meredith and James. There was no way I could make it to Beki and Adam's house. What a shame. I slowly climbed the stairs to spend the day in bed.

Lying in bed with Percy, I drifted in and out of sleep throughout the afternoon. This was what was needed but it was rather sad for me. This is when the Christmas spirit began to shine through. You know, that magical time of year that we try and make last for another 364 days. It all started when I received a phone call from Mark. He was checking in on Percy and me. He asked me to go to the computer as folks were lined up to talk with me on Skype. To my delight, I got to see and talk with all of the children and grandchildren.

Wow! They had organized a way for me to see all of them and join in the fun. To add to the joy, they set a place at the Christmas dinner table for me that they referred to as "Jo-Ann's Place". (Although I heard later they did naughty things with my eating utensils.) And that, for me, was a confirmation that the Christmas spirit is alive and well.

2.7 On Our Way

Sorry about that, Jo-Ann. Not one of my stellar moments. You must agree, though, the kids are creative.

Yes, they certainly are. Don't worry, Percy, a new year is almost here and we're moving along quite nicely. Our new normal is under way and I feel deep down in my bones that we're going to have an amazing year. I think we've arrived at the last three stages of the grieving process. I can see light at the end of the long and dark tunnel.

Hey, I can relate to that.

Percy, really!

Ha ha. Couldn't resist. On a serious note, remind me, please. What are the last three stages of the grieving process again?

Certainly. Number 5 is the upward turn, 6. reconstruction and working through, 7. acceptance and hope. Let's see, my body is having a devil of a time, but we're working hard at making it stronger, so that's an upward turn. We're building a new normal for ourselves and that would fit in nicely with reconstruction and working through. And, well ... Like it or not, it's you and me, Percy, and I know we're hopeful that things will get better and better, in spite of it all. Yup, I really think we've put a lot behind us and we're arriving at acceptance and hope. Now it's off to Florida!

We're going to be in the car for a number of days running; we have approximately 2,620 kilometres (1,628 miles), about a 24-hour drive ahead of us. We plan to drive six to eight hours per day with rest stops added. I'm not sure how Percy and I will endure the long hours and days it will take with me sitting bent at the waist in the passenger seat. Mark prefers to do most of the driving. I'm the navigator with the assistance of the GPS. He needs to not only be alert, he also needs to be stimulated enough not to become drowsy. And so, I think I'll distract myself and entertain Mark with learning and sharing information on the various places we drive through as we head to Naples, Florida. Armed with my fact books and maps, I think the drive will be interesting and informative.

As we begin, the drive is filled with natural beauty and interesting history. Canada is the second largest country in area after Russia, and is slightly larger than the United States, but has a population of only 11 percent as many people as the US. It's one of the least densely populated countries for its size in the world. Most Canadians live within 160 kilometres (100 miles) of the border with the United States.

As an ostomate, when I travel this many hours for that many days, I find wearing clothing that is stiff, such as jean material, with a waistband and zipper, is very uncomfortable. In a sitting position bent at the waist with a waistband is difficult because my original surgery incision and deep scarring run from above my belly button and down from there, and is situated in the middle of my abdomen. Then, of course, Percy sits — as Percy puts it — east southeast of my belly button, with his equipment attached. For me, to sit for long periods of time with stiff material is quite restrictive. For Percy, in particular. And, as mentioned, for the deep abdominal scar tissue. I realized very early on that it is best for me to wear stretchy clothing as this helps alleviate restriction; and there is room for expansion if Percy decides to partake in an unexpected workout. The stretch allows for limited expansion when required, and will hold me over till we can find a facility, stop, park the car, and deal with Percy and his equipment.

I know. I partake at any given time. When I please and how much I please.

Yes, Percy, you're an independent stoma and you flow with the rhythm of our natural digestive clock. And I must say, for the most part, you really don't have a sense of what timing, let alone convenient timing, is.

Oh, yes. Sorry about that, but it is what it is, Jo-Ann. But there are some ostomates who are able to somewhat regulate their movements, aren't there?

Yes. It's called "ostomy irrigation" and it is a way to regulate movements by emptying the colon at a scheduled time. There is a process, equipment, and a personal schedule involved and for many, doing it once a day, or once every second day, the colon can be somewhat trained. Unfortunately, irrigation is not for everyone, only some folks are candidates. An ostomate would need to discuss if this is an option for them with their doctor or an enterostomal nurse who is specially trained. Percy, you and I are not candidates so living with you is always a surprise.

Pardon the pun, but let's get moving, Jo-Ann. We're on our way to Florida.

Absolutely, we're on our way and we've already crossed the Canada–US border. We are now entering the state of New York via the Thousand Islands Bridge, an international bridge system over the St. Lawrence River that connects northern New York with southeastern Ontario in Canada. The actual international border bridge crossing is a set of two parallel 27-metre-long (90-foot) bridges between Hill Island in Canada and Wellesley Island in the United States.

We've entered the United States and we find ourselves in the land of forests, rivers, mountains, lakes, farms and little towns. As we continue along the highway, we are entering what seems to be the land in the clouds with its endless mountains. Up and down, with elevations varying greatly, we navigate high ridges and steep ravines dotted with grassy pasturelands of Upper New York State and into Pennsylvania. The highway brings us through picturesque and scenic vistas that take our breath away. Of course we are driving in winter and we never know when a snow squall will blanket us.

As life would have it on this trip, a snow and ice storm has hit while we are in the mountains and we've come upon multiple cars and trucks that have slid off the highway into the ditches. We're Canadians. We live in a snow belt region of Canada. We are used to these conditions so it's simply slow going and drive on. Mark is an expert in navigating through these conditions and so we move on, as Percy would say.

Still farther we travel to finally arrive at our first overnight stop, which is Harrisburg, Pennsylvania. Harrisburg played a notable role in American history during the American Civil War. Harrisburg was a significant training centre for the Union army, with tens of thousands of troops passing through Camp Curtin and a major rail centre. As a result of this importance, it was a target of General Robert E. Lee's Army of Northern Virginia during its two invasions: the first time during the 1862 Maryland Campaign when Lee planned to capture the city after taking Harpers Ferry, West Virginia, but was prevented from doing so by the Battle of Antietam, and his subsequent retreat back into Virginia; the second attempt was made during the Gettysburg Campaign in 1863 and was more substantial. A short skirmish took place in June 1863 at Sporting Hill, just two miles west of Harrisburg. In addition, Harrisburg was a notable stopping place along the Underground Railroad as escaped slaves being transported across the Susquehanna River were often fed and supplied before heading north toward the northern United States and Canada.

Mark is a history buff, and he is wonderful to travel with through this part of the country that is filled with so much American history. Percy and I are delighted to point out names of towns around and south of Harrisburg, ask a question, then have Mark take it away. We learn so much. For example, when we point out the town of Gettysburg, Mark states: the Battle of Gettysburg, one of the largest battles during the American Civil War, was fought between 1–3 July 1863 across the fields south of the town. Casualties were high; there were over 27,000 Confederate and 31,000 Union losses. The soldiers' bodies are interred at Gettysburg National Cemetery where, on November 19, 1863, Abraham Lincoln attended a ceremony to officially consecrate the grounds and where he delivered his famous Gettysburg Address.

Percy, you're quiet considering we're having to eat food we haven't cooked ourselves, and we don't know what triggers could be in the food. We're fortunate so far. Let's keep up the good work.

Will do.

It's been a long drive today. We've made so much progress. We're safe and it is time to enjoy a good supper. With the miles of mountains, clouds, snow and ice of our day floating through our minds, and as the old stories and songs fill our dream ears, it's time for a good night's sleep.

Night, night, Percy.

Good night, Jo-Ann.

2.8 A Near Miss

Percy.

Yes, Jo-Ann?

You let me sleep all night! No treks to the bathroom. You've been quiet all night. Thanks, little buddy.

You're welcome.

Time to wake up, go for a quick breakfast, and then we'll hit the road again. Soon, the relaxing 4-lane highway of the morning begins to give way to something more hectic. We have entered Maryland. This state is one of the smallest states in terms of area, and it is one of the most densely populated States in the United States. Our fellow drivers are increasing in number and we're conforming to the fast-moving pattern of humanity and their vehicles moving at high speeds all around us.

As we continue on our journey, we enter what is called the "Capital Beltway", a circumferential highway that completely bypasses the District of Columbia and Arlington, cutting a lot of time off our overall drive. According to my map, the Capital Beltway is just over 101 kilometres long (63 miles) with 35 kilometres (22 miles) in Virginia and 65 kilometres (41.7 miles) in Maryland. For the most part, it is eight lanes (four each way) and in time, it will be expanded to ten to twelve lanes in other stretches of the highway.

With vehicles moving to the left of us, to the right of us, in front of us and to the rear, I notice a large white SUV begin to exit off the beltway ramp behind us as we continue straight down the highway. All of a sudden, instead of continuing to drive onto the exit ramp as it had been headed down, the evil four-wheeled antagonist, as though powered by a demonic force, changes its mind about exiting and at the last moment veers to the left, moving right up alongside our car and there isn't much more of a lane in front of it to continue forward. The only way for the demon to continue forward is to force us into the lane to the left of us. The problem is, there are vehicles in that lane so we cannot just simply move over. The SUV now decides, since it is quickly running out of road, that it will stomp on the gas and try to race in front of us. With cars lined up behind us, we cannot slow down fast enough to make room, and to slam on the brakes would cause an accident from behind. It was at this time, looking out my passenger side window, that I saw there was only about 2.5 centimetres (1 inch) between the white demon's mirror and my side mirror.

We have no where to go! A side swipe crash is imminent!

Interestingly, I noticed my hand instinctively go down to my abdomen and I covered Percy. Then, in that fraction of an instant, time slowed down and my thoughts turned to the past couple of years. All the suffering from my disease flashed through my mind and the miracle of survival at the hands of expert doctors. This was followed by thoughts of my struggle to begin and sustain a spectacular recovery, mixed with all my future hopes for a new life for Percy, Mark and me. Then, Chris and Beth's wedding popped into my mind. All of these thoughts flashed through my inner vision and it's some reckless person with his hands on the steering wheel of over a ton of metal, plastic, rubber and horsepower, who decides to change his mind in mid-exit from a busy highway with no room for anyone to manoeuvre, and this is how it ends?

I did not yell, nor did I scream. Mark is a very good driver. He knows what's going on and the last thing he needs is to be distracted and unnerved further by a scream. I closed my eyes, gave thanks for everything and waited for the smash, bangs and crash that as it turned out, never came.

Mark had scanned every possible alternative to avoid a crash and there were none so he simply kept a steady pace and waited for fate to take its course. Either the person would somehow speed up enough on what little of the shoulder of the highway was left to go past us, or the vehicle behind us would notice what was happening and take his or her foot off the accelerator, possibly making just enough room for the white demon. Well, there were very few alternatives as I said, and as it turned out, the demon vehicle realized the folly of trying to speed past us and was able to somehow slow down enough to take a degree of control and eventually merge into the traffic behind us. The quick-thinking driver behind us had obviously done everything he could to avoid an accident by accommodating the demon. Thank you, whoever you are.

Wow, that was a close call, Jo-Ann! Thanks for covering me with your hand. You're my hero. That was a double protection because you already have a special stoma protection device that slips on the seatbelt.

I guess that makes us even, Percy. We both take care of one another.

Just after Percy was created, Mark was concerned for Percy's protection when I wear a seatbelt because Percy is perfectly aligned with the belt as it crosses my lower abdomen. There are many very good products available. The one we decided on secures onto the seatbelt using Velcro and it can be positioned over the stoma. It helps Percy and me enjoy driving without Percy or the pouch being crushed and uncomfortable. It can be left on the seatbelt or be slid off to the side if I'm sharing my vehicle with a passenger. I can also remove it whenever I like and affix it to the driver's seatbelt.

This incident with the white demon is a reminder of how precious and fragile life is in any circumstance, situation, or even on a sunny-day drive down the highway. We're safe for the moment, Florida awaits, and we're still alive to make our date with Chris and Beth's wedding celebration.

Life is good!

2.9 Bluegrass, Revolutionary War & Good Eats

We left the white demon far behind and our next stop was the State of Virginia Welcome Center. Percy and I need to put our feet on the ground and collect ourselves. Whew, that was close. We're hungry so some good eats are also on the agenda.

Virginia is the site of the first English settlement in the United States. In October 1781, the war with the British virtually came to an end when General Cornwallis was surrounded and forced to surrender the British position at Yorktown, Virginia. Two years later, the Treaty of Paris made it official: America was independent. It is also the state where more major battles of the Civil War were fought than any other State.

One of Virginia's many gifts is Bluegrass and Mountain music that has been passed down for generations. Music that finds its roots in Shenandoah [Native word meaning *daughter of the stars*], western Virginia. This lovely State boasts beautiful valleys, lazy rivers, hazy farmland and the Blue Ridge Mountains.

For us, Virginia does not have any snow nor ice on the ground and the bite of the winter is no longer nipping at our heels. Haven't seen any leaves yet on the sycamores, hickories, oaks or maples we are passing as we drive down the interstate, but the hint of greenery is growing more and more apparent. When we started this journey two days earlier, we were immersed in the deep freeze of our home country then, as we travel mile after mile, the winter is melting into green grass and the anticipation of flowers. It is an amazing experience.

The next state we enter is North Carolina. This southeastern state borders South Carolina and Georgia to the south, Tennessee to the west, Virginia to the north, and the Atlantic Ocean to the East. North Carolina has a wide range of elevations, from sea level on the coast to 2,037 metres (6,684 feet) at Mount Mitchell, the highest point in the Eastern US.

We've just passed a highway sign for Fayetteville. Filled with history, the area of Fayetteville was inhabited by various Native American peoples, such as the Eno, Shakori, Waccamaw, Keyauwee and the Cape Fear People. There have been successive cultures of other indigenous peoples in the area for more than 12,000 years. After violent upheavals during the second decade of the eighteenth century, the area was colonized by Scots from Scotland. After the American Revolutionary war, the town was named in honour of General Lafayette, a French military hero who significantly aided the American Army during the war.

The State is known by the nickname "Old North State". I observed references to this name and had to do some research to understand. As it is written, in 1710 the Carolina colony was divided when Edward Hyde was appointed by the Lords Proprietors to be Governor for North Carolina, independent of the Governor of South Carolina. The southern part was called South Carolina and the older, northern settlement, North Carolina. This was when the nickname "Old North State" was born.

The open road continues to beckon us, south ever south.

2.10 Happy, Skippy, Skippy, Do a Little Dance!

Jo-Ann.

Yes, Percy.

I'm really enjoying our journey but I must say, I'm feeling very restricted. I feel like I'm choking.

Oh dear. Hmm ... I hear you, little buddy. Time to make a stop, get out of the car, we have to check your pouch anyway. The timing works well. We've just crossed the border and we're now entering South Carolina. Here's the exit for the Welcome Center. Time to get out of the car and stretch.

Thanks, Jo-Ann.

Happy, happy, skippy, skippy, do a little dance! Daffodils, tulips, hyacinths and crocuses blooming in every flower box! It is official, winter is behind us.

While at the Welcome Center, I learn more about the State of South Carolina. South Carolina is composed of five geographic areas and diverse weather: Outer to Inner Coastal Plains, Deltas, the Blue Ridge Mountains, the Sandhills (ancient dunes from what used to be South Carolina's coast millions of years ago), to South Carolina's present-day coastline that is graced by the Atlantic Ocean. The State boasts natural ports such as Georgetown and Charleston. Of course, there is also the golf mecca of many of our friends and family, Myrtle Beach.

About thirty Native American Groups had lived in what is now South Carolina by the time the first Europeans arrived in the region. It is believed that the first humans settled in current South Carolina about 15,000 years ago.

The first European to land was Francisco Gordillo in 1521, from Spain. Five years later, in 1526, another Spaniard, Lucas Vazquez de Ayllon, founded the first European settlement in the territory that now constitutes the United States. This settlement was named San Miguel de Gualdape and was founded with 600 settlers, including African slaves, but was abandoned three months later. The region would later be claimed by both the Spanish and the French. England claimed the current South Carolina at the beginning of the seventeenth century. In 1629, King Charles I gave the southern colonies to Robert Heath. This colony included the regions that now constitute North Carolina, South Carolina, Georgia and Tennessee. Heath named this colony Carolana, a Latin word which basically means "Land of Charles".

South Carolina has a humid subtropical climate, although high-elevation areas in the Upstate area have less subtropical characteristics than areas on the Atlantic coastline. Coastal areas of the State have very mild winters with highs approaching an average of 16°C (60°F) and overnight lows in the 5–8°C (41–46°F) range. Perfect for the beautiful spring flowers surrounding the Welcome Center. How exquisite!

How are you feeling now Percy?

Feeling much better, Jo-Ann. Let's hit the road.

Great. It's on the road again for us.

2.11 Everything is Peachy

As we cross the border into the State of Georgia, known as the Peach State, the sun is shining and the open road is spread out before us. Historic Georgia was settled in 1733 by James Oglethorpe and was the last of the original 13 Colonies to be formed. Named after King George II of Great Britain, Georgia's true purpose was to be a military buffer zone for the rest of the Colonies from the Spanish in Florida. It officially became a State in 1788.

Georgia bypassed most of the action during the Revolutionary War; however, it became a hotbed of activity during the Civil War, with many important battles taking place within its borders. In 1829, gold was discovered in the North Georgia Mountains, which led to the Georgia Gold Rush. The subsequent influx of White settlers put pressure on the government to take land from the Cherokee Nation. In 1830, President Andrew Jackson signed the Indian Removal Act into law, sending many eastern Native American nations to reservations in present-day Oklahoma. In 1838, Martin Van Buren dispatched federal troops to gather the Cherokee and deport them west of the Mississippi. This forced a relocation known as the Trail Of Tears and which led to the death of over 4,000 Cherokee.

As we drive on, the highway is lined with red cedar, pines, cypress and palmettos. Wow. Palmettos! The first of many palm trees I'm looking forward to enjoying as we head farther south. The road trip continues.

2.12 Gateway to Florida

Palm trees bending with the breeze, flowers in flower boxes, the sun is shining and we've just crossed the border into the State of Florida!

The first Florida city we pass through is Jacksonville, situated in what is referred to as the First Coast region of northeast Florida on the banks of the St. Johns River, and about 40 kilometres (25 miles) south of the Georgia State line, and about 550 kilometres (340 miles) north of Miami. The Jacksonville beaches are adjacent to the Atlantic Ocean coast.

Jo-Ann.

Yes, Percy.

I think I'm feeling a bit off. How much longer do we have to drive today?

Well. We're approximately 575 kilometres (358 miles) from our destination in Naples. Don't worry, Percy, we're not driving all the way to Naples today, we're going to stop for the night in a couple of hours. It's New Year's Eve and we have some celebrating to do tonight!

Not sure how much celebrating I can handle tonight, Jo-Ann.

Oh, dear. I guess all the restaurant meals in the past few days is catching up with us.

Yup.

I'll share a bit more of Florida's history, Percy. That'll keep us going till we stop for the night.

Sure, Jo-Ann, go for it.

The history of Florida can be traced back to when the First Peoples began to inhabit the peninsula as early as 14,000 years ago. They left behind artefacts and archaeological evidence. Written history begins with the arrival of Europeans to Florida; the Spanish explorer Juan Ponce de Leon in 1513. The State was the first mainland realm of the United States to be settled by Europeans. From that time of contact, Florida has had many waves of immigration including French and Spanish settlements during the sixteenth century as well as entry of new Native groups migrating from elsewhere in the south and free Blacks and escaped slaves who became known as Black Seminoles.

Florida was under colonial rule by Spain and Great Britain during the eighteenth and nineteenth centuries before becoming a territory of the United States in 1822. Two decades later, in 1845, Florida was admitted to the union as the 27th US State.

Florida is nicknamed the "Sunshine State" due to its warm climate and days of sunshine. It attracts people like us, and it has become a retirement destination.

How are you feeling now, Percy?

Not good. I'm starting to feel bloated. And there is pain.

Okay, Percy. We just have a short drive to go still. How about I tell you a little about Florida's diverse and amazing ecosystems?

Sure. I need to be distracted right now.

One of the many aspects of Florida Mark and I enjoy are the diverse ecosystems. Within a few miles, and at times within a few inches in altitude, the various species of plants and animals that inhabit its forests, prairies, swamps, lakes, streams and reefs, is incredible. The State has an amazing biodiversity. As I understand it, there are three major ecosystems: Coastal, Fresh Water/Wetlands/Aquatic, and an Upland system.

For anyone who enjoys walking on the beach, Florida's coastal ecosystems are terrific. When we go to the beach, it seems as though people from all over the world join us to play in the sand. We enjoy taking hikes at the various State Parks that protect rookeries of the many birds and animals that inhabit these environmental treasuries. In addition, there are many sea turtles that come from all over the world to lay their eggs on Florida's Atlantic coast. From the sandy shores, we observe pelicans and dolphins. We collect shells for the grandchildren and we watch the sun set over the Gulf of Mexico.

The Fresh Water/Wetlands/Aquatic systems make Florida a State with a lot of aquatic diversity. From the mangroves that prevent erosion, to the swamps and marshes that filter the water naturally, the Everglades for example, these systems have a way of transporting us back to the land before time. It's not unusual to see the American Alligator sunning herself at the edge of the water as the Bald Eagle gracefully circles above. Osprey hunt the waters, as the White Ibis hunts the shoreline.

The Upland systems are divided into two categories: the Florida Pine Flatwoods and the South Florida Flatwoods; both systems are very different from one another. For example, the Pine Flatwoods are interspersed with isolated cypress, marshes, wet prairies, and upland pine scrub. The South Florida Flatwoods are typically savannahs with a sprinkle of grasslands and forest.

We so enjoy Florida not only for the warmth it gives us during the dark and cold winter months, but also for what it provides us in the way of the joy of exploring nature that is so very different from home.

Good news, Percy. We've arrived at the hotel we're staying at for the night.

Thank goodness. Not a moment too soon. We have a lot to look forward to now that we've arrived in Florida and you did distract me with your ... well ... descriptive narrative. But, sheesh. I just really need to explore the chilled tiled floor of the functional hotel bathroom with its fluffy towels so neatly arranged.

Okay, Percy. I get it. We're tired, road weary, and the accumulative affects of the past three days of restaurant food is really getting to us. We need to have a time out.

Unfortunately, there is no real time out for ostomates, nor for any other individual who has an ongoing condition. Although a portion of my large bowel and rectal stump was removed and Percy my stoma was created, some of the underlying conditions that caused the problem in the first place continue. There are many trigger foods that cause Percy and me a lot of digestive issues. For example, I am very sensitive to food additives such as artificial colouring, preservatives, flavourings ... and the list goes on. Other ostomates will have their own set of trigger foods. Bottom line here: having a chronic condition doesn't necessarily mean an illness is critical. Some chronic conditions like having irritable bowel, colitis, Crohn's, asthma, arthritis, diabetes, etc., come with underlying conditions. Even when a person feels healthy some of the time, they will have to deal with symptoms to be endured. And so, as we say goodbye to the old year and ring in the new year, Percy, Mark and I will deal with the ravages of Percy's latest poonami as best we can.

2.13 Florida Fun

With last evening's poonami and many miles behind us, we're now settled in our Naples, Florida digs. The sun is shining and the air is warm. Hallelujah!

I can now wear sandals exposing my psoriasis hands and feet to the air, and I do hope this will help the skin on my heels. If nothing else, going without socks and closed-in shoes will give me some relief.

Every morning as I take my long walk, the drop foot slows me down so I'm very careful navigating any speed bumps in the hopes that I don't end up head over heels.

We stop at local farmers' markets to purchase juicy and scrumptious fresh fruits and vegetables. This is definitely going to help build my body strength, giving me an added boost in preparation for the upcoming surgery.

Florida for me at this time is about gaining strength physically, emotionally, mentally and nourishing my human spirit. I've decided I will tuck the thought of the upcoming surgery away into a dark and not-often-used part of my mind for the time being and just get on with the healthy living of the moment.

As the lazy hazy days pass by, there is the business of finding a dress to wear to Beth and Chris's wedding, which I have decided I will purchase in Florida. I am excited and, of course, apprehensive as I have to cover what may or may not be a lopsided body by the time of the wedding. As I don't know how the surgery will go and what my abdominal profile will be,

I simply have to find something that will work for every eventuality.

Oh, me ... me ...

Percy, what would you like to say?

I would like to share our shopping adventure with everyone.

Of course, Percy, go right ahead.

I like to call this little shopping story of ours "Percy Gets A New Dress". Here we are in sunny Florida, basking in the warmer-than-usual southwest Florida weather. Meanwhile, our family and friends at home are navigating snow-covered roads, bracing themselves against a − 31°C (− 23°F) wind-chill factor. Do wish everyone could be here with us.

Southwest Florida is known for sunshine, Everglades, white sand beaches and some of the best bargain hunting outlets we've ever come across. With Beth's wedding scheduled for the end of June, what better place to shop for a dress?

Now it must be understood that Jo-Ann is not a happy camper when shopping even at the best of times. It's just not her thing. That's when she asks her sister-in-law, Nola, to join her. Nola has a great fashion sense, loves shopping, is very patient, and is gently honest with what suits and what does not. So it's off with Nola to shop.

Jo-Ann and Nola's mission, if they choose to accept it, is to find a step-mother-of-the-bride dress that will suit Jo-Ann and camouflage me while getting as much bang for her buck as possible. It was early morning — the early bird gets the worm — and already it was hot and steamy. With the GPS on the car dash, Nola and Jo-Ann leave for the outlet.

We parked the car and took a reconnoitre of the vast parking lot, already beginning to fill, and got a sense of the lay of the land. Across the horizon, as far as we could see, there were stores, stores, and more stores.

Nola was excited to get started and Jo-Ann was almost overwhelmed. Our first stop was the outlet map. X marked the spot where we were standing and it was time to get moving.

Like a river running through a canyon, we walked the ribbon of concrete between store fronts. Buildings to our right and to our left. We were three on a quest for the perfect dress. I am situated on top of a honey-dew-melon-sized parastomal hernia on the left side of Jo-Ann's abdomen. There are times when she's aware of her lopsided physique.

Under Nola's expert guidance, somewhat timid Jo-Ann gained confidence and started to feel rather MacGyver-ish. There are resourceful fashion solutions. It's simply a matter of fashion awareness. Jo-Ann realized that she now must consider and in some cases change, her fashion style. Clothing that she has liked before, for the most part, do not suit her new body shape. How to do this? Well, time to consider what draws the eye to other more flattering body parts. Next, find clothing that is constructed in such a way as to draw the eye to a decorative focal point such as a strategically placed buckle, pleats, and so on.

Looking at various fabric prints, Jo-Ann realized there are patterns with various colour palettes that create a general look that once again pulls the eye with pleasing results. And finally, Jo-Ann has learned to stay away from fabrics that cling.

It was time to enter the cool and brightly lit stores. Splitting up to cover as much ground as possible, Jo-Ann and I went to one set of racks, and Nola to another. As I mentioned, I'm situated on the left side, and so my camouflage requires strategic placement there. As our quest continued under the hot mid-morning sun, Nola would find a nice dress that might suit. Jo-Ann would try it on, only to realize that the focal point of that particular dress would be on the opposite side of me.

Personally, my lumpy profile with a flower on the opposite side seems quite interesting to me but Jo-Ann and Nola certainly didn't think so. I can't tell you how many times we did this. Nola would hold up a dress and say "hey, this one looks great, oh it's right handed", and they would chuckle. Store staff even got into it with them, being very helpful and understanding. Jo-Ann would say "see my right side profile, this is what I look like. Now, see my left side profile, this is what I really look like." A small army of determined women in each of the stores joined us on our quest. And then the moment we all anticipated arrived. Nola found a deep purple velvet dress. It has pleats that fold diagonally from the right across the bodice and down the dress to the waist. It all meets on the left, coming together with a chiffon material that gathers into what reminds me of a flower. From the flower, the material becomes a vertical wave of wide ribbons of chiffon that drape down to almost the hem line. The dress is elegant.

With a bit of a flare, it accentuates Jo-Ann's assets and camouflages me.

Three cheers, high fives and a hip hip hurray. Our mission is a success! Our quest has been fulfilled with all the twists, turns, challenges and camaraderie a shopping trip offers. Our last stop is the cash register.

At home, we guesstimate the dress would probably cost us in the $200-Canadian-range. But we are at a South Florida outlet where sales abound so who knew what the last press of the cash register's screen would reveal. Jo-Ann held her breath. Nola winked as they waited for the final sale.

With a smile on her face, the store representative announced, "That, will be $18.50."

Jo-Ann and Nola looked at the register's digital screen. Yes. The electronic print read $18.50. Astounding, incredible, amazing were the thoughts that passed through Jo-Ann's mind. These thoughts translated into giggles, laughs, and a few OMGs.

As with any successful quest in life, there is always something to be learned and this one was not an exception. I learned, with a little sense — in this case fashion sense — and with some resourcefulness and commitment, that all people are beautiful just the way we are, including me, just as I am.

Percy, that was great story telling, thanks.

I love the dress. When I put it on and look at myself in the mirror, the question that comes to mind is, "Stoma what stoma?"

As the days and weeks progress, in spite of the various daily physical issues I have to deal with, my general health is terrific and my worries are hidden away for the time being. We're playing in the sunshine, life is good, and I have my camera in hand.

I just can't get over the fact we live on such a beautiful planet. Our home is a wondrous place filled with drama and visual splendour. An interesting subject will appear, a contrast of light and shadow will become apparent, or a drama will unfold. This is when I focus and snap. A life image and an Earth moment in time is captured to be enjoyed and relived over and over again.

Percy and I get a real kick out of taking our camera just about everywhere we can, hunting for great photographic shots. Life never ceases to show up as we delight in snapping away the day. Once again, the magic of life showed up on our day trip to Marco Island, Florida. We were waiting to board the *Marco Island Princess* for a sunset cruise and it was a very breezy day. Looking over my shoulder, I spotted a Snowy Egret clinging to a railing and holding on for dear life.

Her feathers were blowing this way and then that way. A bad-feather day would be an understatement. I slowly and carefully walked up to her, camera in my hand, and then snapped. We captured her moment. So as to not stress her any more than she must have been experiencing, I took one more quick photo and then quickly walked away giving her as wide a berth as possible so she could do something, anything, to stay upright on the railing and tame her ruffled feathers. Some of us know what that's like first thing in the morning.

I call this photograph, "Bad Feather Day", and it sure makes me smile, chuckle and ponder. This Snowy Egret is the gift of humour and steadfastness for me, and she's also metaphor. Throughout our lives the winds of hardship blow from time to time, threatening to push us over and slam us to the ground. Yet even with the odds seemingly against us, most of us hang in there, even when it's about hanging on for dear life. All of us who have had a second chance at life know this. Our feathers are ruffled, so to speak, as we lean in, and we weather the storms. Our drive to live and get on with getting on with life is intense, even in the most challenging of times.

We don't know when or if the winds will cease. With all the strength and will we have within, we and our support system (if we are lucky enough to have one), grasp and cling onto the most solid and steady thing we can. Being a human is not for wimps! Hurrah to all who choose to live a joyous and the fullest of lives, in spite of it all.

No matter our life situations, we all have hopes and dreams and during a lifetime, harsh winds will blow from time to time. Like the seemingly delicate Snowy Egret, we are amazingly strong even on our worst bad-feather day.

(For more information about fashion for ostomates, go to "Information, Tips & Hints" section.)

2.14 Percy Blasts Off

Now Percy has a new dress. We've been in Florida for the past six weeks and I'm so happy Percy has, for the most part, been a cooperative little stoma. The next chapter of our life story is about to begin, and I think we're going to celebrate this by taking the day to visit Kennedy Space Center, which is located on what is called the Space Coast of Florida (Atlantic Ocean side). I feel it's important to share this adventure as it was such a wonderful experience; but it also was an experience whereby in my inexperience at having an ostomy could have seriously injured Percy.

As the promotional material states: "For the last 50 years, Kennedy Space Center has been the gateway to space exploration", it is the launch site of space science and discovery. Our day began with multiple cinematic journeys to the end of the Earth and beyond. First, we embarked on a visual and sensory three-dimensional adventure of our world that transported us beyond Earth. Together we explored the Solar System.

With the end of a cosmic adventure through our galactic neighbourhood, it was then off to the IMAX theatre. We gazed at the Hubble space telescope in 3-D, on a five-storey movie screen. Oh, my. Mark, Percy and I, were transported through the beautiful and mysterious Universe.

From the amazing "out there", we returned closer to home as we viewed the Space Station 3-D film. From planet Earth to the International Space Station, we enjoyed the movie that was filmed by twenty-five astronauts and cosmonauts. We were amazed.

All of these experiences filled our imaginations with endless possibilities, fuelling our desire to experience space for ourselves. We wanted to see what an astronaut sees and feel what they feel. It was time to know what it's like to be launched into orbit at 17,500 mph!

Feeling quite courageous, we embarked on our Shuttle Launch. We were directed to a wall of equipment lockers by the staff. Here I stowed my backpack which includes Percy's back-up ostomy equipment. (I always carry this in case of a poop emergency.) This should have been my first clue.

From here we were directed into a building with a huge multi-screen wall. We were put through an 8½-minute "pre-flight" briefing presented by astronaut Charlie Bolden, which was designed for the purpose of preparing us for lift off. That should have been my second clue.

It was time for the experience of a lifetime. We and our fellow shuttle-launch team left the pre-flight room and lined up in our respective lines awaiting the shuttle ride doors to open.

Capable and helpful Shuttle guides reminded the team that people with medical conditions — expectant mothers and so on — were welcome to experience the shuttle launch from a special room that presented all the sights and sounds of the launch, but without the physical part of the launch. Clue number three.

For the rest of us, we were congratulated and reminded we were about to experience the sights, sounds, feelings and excitement of a vertical launch in humankind's most complex vehicle. We were about to live the thrilling launch experience of an astronaut crew aboard NASA's Space Shuttle. Clue number four.

Now it was our turn to see what they have seen, feel what they have felt, and live what they have lived.

The doors opened and we embarked into the simulation Shuttle cockpit. Rows of folks walked into the ship and we sat in our seats. As you would find on a roller coaster ride, large metal security bars framed each seat, and we were instructed to secure our seat belts.

I reached down and buckled my seat belt, and this is when I realized the belt was located right over my parastomal hernia and Percy! This is something I had not thought of and now I had a problem. How would Percy endure the Shuttle launch?

I pulled the belt lower down over my abdomen and below Percy. The belt snapped right back up over Percy. I pulled the belt up above Percy and it snapped back over Percy. Percy was caught in a situation that I had not anticipated, and I started to worry. I had put my little buddy in a potentially harmful situation.

The launch was about to begin and my thoughts were with Percy. It was countdown time. I quickly slipped both my hands down under the seatbelt and cupped Percy in them, hoping to protect him.

10 – 9 – 8 – 7 – 6 – 5 – 4 – 3 – 2 – 1 BLAST OFF

The noise level escalated, the visuals raced before my eyes, and the definite, yet certainly not overly violent, shake, rattle and slight roll began. With both hands surrounding Percy, we began to immerse ourselves into the most extraordinary and wonderful experience. With the exception of feeling the g-forces, the launch was everything we hoped it would be.

When the launch simulation ended, I released my hands and quickly unbuckled the seat belt. Percy seemed none the worse for wear. Excited, I headed for the toilet facilities for a more in-depth Percy inspection. He was absolutely fine.

I do feel my wild days of riding the roller coaster are now over, but I fully expect to enjoy more tame types of rides though. The Shuttle launch was our first experience of its kind since Percy's creation. Gee ... Ostomies affect all aspects of an ostomate's life. I did not think of the seat belt and Percy's placement, and it is a good lesson to learn.

Percy and I wear our seatbelt in the car at all times. I now realize how important it is that I disconnect the seatbelt ostomy protection equipment and bring it with me for any eventuality when enjoying rides.

Most important lesson: As long as I am vigilant of Percy's needs, have the foresight to analyze situations, know/accept our limitations, and be resourceful. We will continue on our quest to live life to the fullest. We choose to live the inspired ostomate's life. Ostomates have already beaten the odds and are living proof of courage. Now that's an adventure of a lifetime.

PART 3

Don't Be Afraid

3.0 On the Road Again

My physical batteries are charged. We are embarking on our journey home, and all of the uncertainly this brings. The ribbons of highway that lie ahead of us are twisted and knotted with bitter/sweet emotions. The compass of my soul is pointing to my north home star, to the golden opportunity to heal some more. But my nerves are shattered at the moment because my mind dwells on the many worst-case surgery and recovery scenarios that could possibly happen. My human sprit is shining with optimism, I know this because deep down I hear a strong voice repeating the mantra, "GET UP. STAND UP. DON'T GIVE UP THE FIGHT!"

We pass the borders of each and every US State as we retrace our steps home. I am confused and conflicted. Hmm ... Each State? It just dawned on me that this is an interesting metaphor for the state I'm physically, emotionally and mentally dwelling in right now. Each separate and at the same time integral.

Jo-Ann.

Yes, Percy.

You know when you get nervous and feel anxiety, it really affects me.

Goodness yes, Percy. I hear you. Well actually, I feel you. You're very sensitive. In fact, medical science has an explanation for what's happening with us.

We as humans have a rather independent nervous system that is referred to as the enteric nervous system (ENS), also known as the intrinsic nervous system. My understanding from research is: the enteric nervous system in our bellies consists of a mesh-like system of neurons that governs the function of the gastrointestinal system. There is a new and surprising view of how the enteric nervous system in our bellies goes far beyond just processing the food we eat.

Everyone, even the steeliest of us, is likely to experience that familiar feeling of "butterflies" in the stomach. Underlying this sensation is the neuron lining of our gut that is so extensive, some scientists have nicknamed it our "second brain".

As I researched further, a deeper understanding of this mass of neural tissue came to light: it is understood that filled with important neurotransmitters, this system seems to do much more than merely handle digestion, or inflict the occasional nervous pang. The little brain in our innards, in connection with the big one in our skulls, partly determines our mental state and plays key roles in certain diseases throughout the body. Although its influence is far-reaching, the second (little) brain is not the seat of any conscious thoughts or decision-making.

The second little brain consists of sheaths of neurons embedded in the walls of the long tube of our gut, starting from the food that enters our bodies and the solid wastes that are expelled. This includes the mouth, pharynx, esophagus, stomach, small intestine, large intestine, and anus.

The second little brain contains some 100 million neurons, more than in either the spinal cord or the peripheral nervous system. This multitude of neurons in the system enables us to "feel" the inner world of our gut and its contents. And so, equipped with its own reflexes and senses, the second little brain can control gut behaviour independently of the big brain.

We are given to understand that our bodies likely evolved this intricate web of nerves to perform digestion and excretion "on site", rather than remotely from our brains through the middleman of the spinal cord. Our bodies relieve the big brain from the messy business of digestion as this is delegated to the brain in the gut.

Some researchers state that the system is way too complicated to have evolved only to make sure things move out of our colon, says Emeran Mayer, professor of physiology, psychiatry and biobehavioral sciences at the David Geffen School of Medicine at the University of California, Los

Angeles (U.C.L.A.). For example, scientists were shocked to learn that about 90 percent of the fibres in the primary visceral nerve are carrying information from the gut to the brain and not the other way around.

The second little brain informs our state of mind in other more obscure ways, as well. "A big part of our emotions are probably influenced by the nerves in our gut," Mayer says. Butterflies in the stomach — signalling in the gut as part of our physiological stress response — is but one example. Turmoil can very well sour our stomachs and our moods.

Cutting-edge research in the field of neurogastroenterology is currently investigating how the second little brain mediates the body's immune response; after all, at least 70 percent of our immune system is aimed at the gut to expel and kill foreign invaders.

U.C.L.A.'s Mayer is doing work on how the trillions of bacteria in the gut "communicate" with the enteric nervous system cells. His work with the gut's nervous system has led him to think that in coming years, psychiatry will need to expand to treat the second little brain in addition to the big one atop the shoulders.

So, Percy, after learning about this, I'm sure going to pay more heed to my so-called "gut feelings" from now on. And I do understand that when I'm upset, it upsets you, too.

Thanks. You know, Jo-Ann, from 2008 to 2011, I was connected in an airless world of pain and illness, and your life force was slipping away. In July of 2011, I was brought out to the light and became partially disconnected and your stoma, where I reside now outside of you and yet I am a life-sustaining part of you. Since 2011 to date, we've lived a lifetime of joy and at the same time we felt that we have died a thousand deaths. A lot of water has passed under that second-chance-at-life bridge. Your perception of your self and life has been altered. This achievement wasn't yours alone, this was also the achievement of your life partner and caregiver, Mark, and the doctors, nurses, your family, friends, and me.

That's so very true, Percy.

Your life has come a long way since the first pangs of pain and discomfort. And now, hundreds of thousands of experiences, episodes, and steps backwards and forward have been experienced as you navigate through another world for the second time in your history. These were and are momentous times for us — extraordinary — for the coordination of your mind and emotions in addition to the skills of the many who made all of this possible. A lot of hard work by you yourself, many others, and me, I might add, has culminated in this moment suspended in time. A moment that has the potential to take your life along a radically different course, come what may. I'm asking you to listen to that mantra, "GET UP. STAND UP. DON'T GIVE UP THE FIGHT!"

Wow, Percy, you have a way of putting things into perspective. Thank you. Your second little brain sure is as sharp as a tack.

3.1 Ready or Not, Here We Come

We arrived home in February and our vacation suitcases are unpacked. The refrigerator and freezer are now re-stocked.

Percy.

Yes, Jo-Ann.

After all of the hurry up and wait, I think the pace is going to pick up.

Are you ready, Jo-Ann?

Ha, ready or not here we come, Percy!

A couple of days after we arrived home, I heard several public service notice announcements on the radio. March is Colorectal Cancer Awareness Month. Although colorectal cancer is not the reason for the creation of my ostomy, there are so many ostomates who have suffered this terrible disease, won the war against it, and are now a part of the fellowship of the bag.

Colorectal cancer remains the second leading cause of cancer deaths in Canada. Approximately one in thirteen Canadian men and one in sixteen Canadian women will be diagnosed with this disease in their lifetime. Individuals can live with colorectal cancer long before they experience any physical symptoms. Both early detection and treatment are key to increasing survival rates.

Colorectal Cancer Awareness Month encourages a dialogue about this disease while aiming to empower people aged 50 to 70 to talk to their doctor about getting screened. While each life that has been lost to colorectal cancer is one too many, at this time, rates have been on the decline in Canada since 2000. The Colorectal Cancer Awareness Month public service notices encourage people to learn more about prevention and testing, as well as services and programs in their community.

We've enjoyed two days of relaxation and the phone rings!

"This is she. Oh, I have a pre-op appointment at the hospital March 8. Yes, we'll be there at 7:30 a.m. Yes, we'll arrive at least 15 minutes beforehand. Yes, I'll have all my necessary papers, health card, hospital card, and a list of medications and vitamins. Do you have a surgery date for me? No? Okay. Thanks. We'll see you then."

Oh, Percy. It has begun! OMG, Percy. It's really going to happen. I'm so nervous. I'm shaking all over and my skin just got really itchy!

Yes, I know, Jo-Ann. Pull yourself together because we need to get to the bathroom, right now, quick!

3.2 The Mute Silence of Anxiety

While attending our pre-op appointment, we spent three hours at the hospital speaking with the admitting nurse and an anaesthetist. I provided my blood for analysis. All the while, we anxiously waited to hear our surgery date. I signed the consent forms after reading all of the things that can go wrong. Oh, that was interesting, to say the least. Next, I was given booklets: *Guide — Planning for My Inpatient Surgery, Guide — Pain Management after Surgery, Welcome to the Hospital Admission Information.* Percy, Mark and I are informed, educated, and prepared.

"I don't have a date written here on the form. Give me a few minutes, and I'll make a call," said the admitting nurse. A few minutes later she returned, "No, we don't have a date yet. I can't tell you when it will be, but do know it will be soon. Meanwhile, avoid anyone with a cold, cough, sniffles, or the flu. You'll be getting a call."

So here we are, still and again, sitting by the phone awaiting the call. I've packed my hospital bag and it stands at the ready. When the phone call does come, I believe things will move very quickly. Percy, Mark and I need to be ready.

Every time the phone rings, we jump! I have informed friends and family I cannot be exposed to any of their potential coughs, sniffles and sneezes.

I've put the phone volume at its loudest, just in case it rings and I'm in the shower. I've cancelled restaurant dates with friends, to protect my health.

Oh for Pete's sake, the phone seems to be ringing constantly and everyone and anyone who is not from the hospital nor my surgeon's office is calling!

Jo-Ann.

Yes, Percy.

Patience!

Doing my best Percy.

That's it. I'm inviting my cough-less, sniffle-less, and sneeze-less friends and family into the, as germ free as possible, confines of my home. I'm no longer concerned I will catch a cough from anyone. I'm more concerned that I'm going to catch a full blown case of cabin fever!

I thought the hurry up and wait would be history by now. I'm sitting here with time on my hands and that means I have too much time to think, to feel, to muse. The anxiety is growing inside me, and I don't want to complain to anyone as they are all on pins and needles with us and they don't need to have to placate me.

During one of my musing moments, youngest daughter (Meredith Henderson) of our blended family, who is an actress, comes to mind. I am always fascinated when I'm with her on set for a movie or for one of her television series sets. Since the only job I have at those times is to observe, then observe is what I do. I am amazed to watch the drama and non-drama of hurry up and wait as it plays out before my eyes.

Off to the side and in the dark corners at-the-ready for action, the production crew members patiently watch the director and actors do their part. When it is time to change the scene and/or location, the crew scramble in a flurry of coordinated activity to prepare and to get everything ready to shoot the next scene of the production.

This is the stage on which I have watched the hurry up and wait dance performed. It is not simple, it is coordinated, specific and very patient theatre. It is one of life's living truths, and there's a good lesson hidden in the scene that I am trying to learn.

It's my turn to dance the patience dance as I wait by the phone, avoiding the coughs, sniffles and sneezes as best I can. And, when it does ring, I will *arabesque* to the phone. I will *assemblé* as they give me the date and time of the surgery. Until then I will *attitude croisé devant* as I *ballon* and *ballotté* my best patience dance steps.

Well, that's the plan at any rate.

3.3 Percy Gets a Facelift

The phone rang earlier today, and our date with destiny has been announced. It is official! I'm nervous and filled with anxiety about what is going to transpire and how Percy and I will get through it. The last surgery I endured was a last-ditch effort to save my life. Everything had gone wrong leading up to the surgery and my spectacular recovery has been a long and drawn out journey that still has not transitioned to a full recovery. We have to prepare ourselves emotionally. We cannot dwell on what could go wrong. I have to bring my human spirit back on track. Oh my, I've got the jitters.

Yeah, I can feel it too, Jo-Ann. To help us get on track, why don't you share what the surgery will actually entail.

Sure, Percy.

Our amazing and incredibly skilful oncologist/surgical-scientist, Dr. Auer, who was the lead when I was carved into a survivor and who had created Percy, will be performing this upcoming surgery. I have so much confidence in her abilities and her amazing bedside manner. She's already saved my life. I feel I'm in good hands. During one of our appointments, she had explained to me she would be performing the "Modified Sugarbaker Technique". She has assured me it is safe and has a low peristomal hernia recurrence rate.

Basically, and in lay terms, our honey-dew-sized lump will undergo an interesting procedure: the intestine will be repacked back in place, abdominal wall muscles will be repaired, and a bio-mesh will be placed in the abdomen in order to support the abdominal wall. Then, to deal with Percy's prolapsed situation, a mesh hammock will be placed around the stoma, this will be done in the hopes it will provide Percy with the stability and support my little buddy requires.

Ha, Percy. You're going to be quite the lazy one resting in your little hammock for the rest of your days.

Lucky me, I'm getting a facelift and I get to swing in my hammock.

Oh dear, I just can't sit still. I'm bouncing all over the place. Time to get myself organized and ready for the big day.

3.4 Best Laid Plans of Mice & Men

There goes the phone, it's ringing again!

"Yes, hello, Nancy," I said to the surgeon's assistant.

"Oh yes, the surgery date is changed, oh dear. Oh, it's been moved up! It's now scheduled for March 19. Okay, we're ready. Report at the same time at the Admittance Desk at 8:00 a.m., certainly. Surgery will be at 1:00 p.m., works for me. Yes, I'll rest and take it easy. Bye."

Percy, it's happening sooner! I'm so nervous. I'm shaking all over and my skin just got really itchy again!

It's party time, Jo-Ann!

What?

It's party time!

Really, Percy?

Hey, we've got four days to major surgery, let the countdown begin. We're ready for the next stage of our healing journey. Let's spend as much time as possible partying with our friends and family. Well, as I like to say: let's be happy and go with the flow.

Not a bad idea, Percy.

Percy and I are ready. We've been given the grand gift of life. The journey and the community of humanity who have shared it with us so far have made the adventure an amazing experience. We are survivors and with this comes a great depth of realization. My near-death experience was the apex of one speck in time, and from that day forward this has given me the opportunity to see life and death for what they are, in all their mysteries and intricate interrelations. For the past few years, Percy and I have had the vantage point from which we've looked over the landscape of our existence; we have seen the line between life and death and it is definitely defined and marked.

As I think back over the past few years, the theme of life and death has run through my mind so very many times. I have lived the duality. I have come to know what that means in my daily life, and also in the grand scheme of my life. According to the dictionary, duality means: instance of opposition or contrast between two concepts — a dualism. As an artist and a photographer, I often capitalize on the dualities of light and dark; and at other times, on stillness and movement. In my life before and after Percy was created, I realize that I am a force of nature that can cease to exist at any given time, and certainly not necessarily at a time of my own choosing. I strive to live and I desire quality of life. I have engaged in celebrations for the life that was my past, and for my second chance at life, my new normal. It's interesting that as mere humans we want to live, we reject death, yet, in truth, we cannot have one without the other. There is no life without death, and there is no death without life. I am filled with anxiety as I think over the major surgery happening in a few days, and the thoughts of what could go wrong are dancing in my head, as any surgery is a risk. Since the onset of the original disease that brought me to the brink, I have felt there has been a magic ingredient in my life. As time and experience have passed, I've come to realize what that special ingredient is for me, and it is determination. Determination to go beyond survival to thriving. I want to express who I am through my thoughts, words and actions for as long as I can, even if I have only a few minutes, hours or days to do so.

Percy and I have worked hard to adjust to our new normal. I must admit when I look at Percy, which is multiple times a day, the little stoma reminds me of some of the lousy life happenings I've had to, and continue to, experience. On the other hand, Percy is my ticket to life. Without Percy, I no longer exist. Talk about duality!

Without Percy, I would not have had the opportunity to witness and enjoy the weddings of the past couple of years, and I would not have leaped with joy with the birth of grandchildren. I would not have been touched by the love of my life partner, and ... and ... and ... and all of the amazing life experiences I've had the pleasure, displeasure, joy, heartache, frustrations and ongoing dualities of experiencing as my life unfolds.

Life can be so confusing and downright difficult with all of its ups and downs, ins and outs, successes and failures. Some of the experiences of the past few years have been so very good and some have been so very bad. As frightened as I am at the thought of the surgery at this time, I think the key to my version of surviving and stepping beyond to thrive is to know a duality when I see it and to make the time that I do have a celebration of life!

So, Percy. Let's party on, dude!

3.5 I Am So Rich, I Am So Grateful

Wouldn't you know it, the big day is tomorrow, and 10 to 20 cm (approximately 4 to 8 inches) of snow is predicted. Stormy weather is pressing in on the Ottawa Valley as the pressure of surgery presses in on us.

Having a somewhat restless night, we in fact did wake up in the morning to a grey sky and swirling snow. One last shower and full body scrub-up which will have to last me for a while, and a few love snuggles with my little cat, Niki. Then, after a curl up in the warmth of his embrace, Mark and I took a few wordless moments with each other. He picked up my suitcase with carefully packed toiletries for the hospital stay, and it was off into the silvery mass of snow.

We arrived at the hospital's admittance office, signed forms and it was off to the pre-op location. My son, Richard, arrived to be with Mark, Percy and me. The staff offered to provide me with medication to relax and semi-sedate me, which I refused. Percy and I are just fine now. We've gone through all the physical and psychological preparation possible for us so now it is time to embrace my human spirit as we step forward and allow our life to unfold as it will.

As I'm a naturally jovial person, the jokes and giggles began flying around my curtained enclosure. All the while, as I lay on the hospital gurney, I gazed at my two amazing and special men. Richard, the now young man I had known since his first spark of life. The little fella who had curled up in my heart and made it grow and glow. The young boy that taught me so very many life lessons through his suffering, attitude, example, successes, strengths and wisdom. The boy who was never supposed to walk as other folks do yet who learned to skip and run. The teenager who became stricken with Crohn's disease, and whom we have almost lost three times because of it, and who has made spectacular comebacks each and every time. The young man who had to endure the grieving process at the unexpected death of his father, at such a young age. The man who, as a child, had always told his daddy and me so many years ago how he was going to have his own family, and who is now a loving husband and a wonderful dad. His wish has come true. I am so rich, I am so grateful, and come what may, I am graced and I'm ready for whatever lies ahead for me.

My gaze shifts over to my husband, Mark, who, at one time, was the young man that I met when I was 17 years of age. The best man for my late husband, Robert, and me when we married so very long ago. The music man who is a song writer, singer and accomplished musician. The father who has supported and nurtured the talents of his four beautiful children as they perform their musical and acting magic on stage, on television, and in film. The then young man who rushed out in the dead of winter without his boots and winter coat and drove for hours in the snow to be with and to support Robert and me when our eldest son suddenly passed away.

The older man who was there for my son, Richard, and me as we grieved Robert's passing. The man who was there for his widow friend and eventually fell in love with this old girl. The man who asked me to marry him in the winter of our lives and has endured my illness, Percy, my recovery, and now my surgery again. He is my husband, my caregiver, and all-round best bud. I am so rich, I am so grateful, and come what may I am graced and I'm ready for whatever lies ahead for me.

"They're here. It's time. Bye, Richard. Love you, honey. Bye, Mark. Love you, sweetheart. Percy and I are ready. We're in good hands. We'll be just fine. See you later. Love you guys whole bunches."

As they wheel my gurney out of the pre-op area and down the hall, I'm relaxed and ready for anything. Little did Percy and I know *anything* would take on a very different flavour than what we could have anticipated as we arrived in the operating theatre.

3.6 Percy Has Star Quality

As I lay on the gurney, watching the ceiling tiles whiz by, the orderly wheeled me down the hospital corridor. Eventually she tucked me close to the wall of the hallway where the bank of operating theatres are located. The young woman stated that it would not be too long and a doctor would come to see me. As I looked around, I realized, without a doubt, that I was in fact in the operating theatre wing. Staff were still in the process of cleaning out one of the operating rooms as I lay there. To my left were steel shelves and on those shelves were the soiled linens removed from a previous surgery. For someone who is not used to viewing this, I must say it was most unpleasant.

Percy!

Yes, Jo-Ann.

I'm getting the jitters again.

I know. Jo-Ann. I'm rattled, too. Won't be long now. We'll be okay. I think.

As I gently patted little Percy, two young resident doctors arrived. The Ottawa Hospital is a teaching hospital which offers primary (general), secondary (specialized) and tertiary (most advanced) health care services. Therefore, residents and fellows who are medical doctors taking specialized training in a particular field will assist an attending physician and collaborate with team members who assist in the patient's treatment. They may also visit the patient every day, plan treatment, and meet with the patient's attending physician to discuss care and treatment.

"Hello, Mrs. Tremblay." They both chimed in together.

"Hello. Just call me Jo-Ann."

"And this is Percy," I said as I patted Percy.

"Yes, Jo-Ann. We know Percy."

At the time, I did not question why they said they knew Percy. I just thought they knew I have a stoma.

"We will be assisting in the surgery today," they said in unison.

"Oh, that's nice," I responded as I tried to find some interesting thing to say.

With my eyes now diverted from the steel shelving, I focused my attention on the doctors. They explained a little about what was going to be happening in a few minutes. They helped me understand that it would be rather chilly in the room, and that there would be many folks moving about in the room preparing for the surgery. They explained that there would be many pieces of equipment, some large and some small. They were providing me with important information, all delivered with gentle and soothing voices. I began to relax. A bit.

Then my gurney started moving and we were on our way!

As I entered the operating theatre, the chilly air temperature slapped me in the face immediately. My eyes scanned the room and the equipment looked very impressive and extremely intimidating to me. I felt my whole body stiffen and all I wanted to do was climb off the gurney, stand up, and then run like heck.

Percy!

I'm scared, too. Remember we have to do this, Jo-Ann. We have too many health risks going on so it is better to get this done now while we're healthy and not when we are in a crisis situation and we're back at the brink again.

Yeah, I know, little buddy. Wait a minute ... Percy. People have stopped moving around. They're all standing and their beautiful faces seem to be greeting us.

Keep talking to me. Jo-Ann. I need to know what's going on.

Well as I mentioned, they have stopped what they were doing and they are all looking at us. Their faces are bright. They all seem to be smiling at us, and their energy feels like open arms that are embracing us. Oh no, Percy. I know they are Earth Angels to be sure, but I hope they're not doing this because they don't think we'll make it, and they're showing us their final respects!

Get a grip, Jo-Ann.

"Hello, Jo-Ann," said one of the Earth Angels in the room.

"I'm your anaesthetist, and I understand we have a celebrity in our midst," she stated with warm enthusiasm.

"Oh my, you treat your patients with such high regard," I responded.

"Yes, everyone is important and precious," she said as a couple of the other Earth Angels helped lift me from the gurney onto the hard, cold metal surface of the operating table.

"I've read your book and I really enjoyed it," she continued.

"Oh, really?"

"Yes. Your surgical oncologist read *Better WITH a Bag than IN a Bag* and she shared it with us. I really enjoyed it, too."

Jo-Ann.

Yes, Percy.

I'm a star.

Yes, Percy. You sure are.

It was at this time that many of the remaining Earth Angels in the room nodded their heads in agreement, gave a quick smile, and then turned back to their surgery preparations, including the anaesthetist who began to explain what she was doing and that within seconds Percy and I would be asleep.

Percy, it'll be seconds now. Hang in there. I'll do the best from my end. Thanks for everything, little buddy.

You too, Jo-Annnnn ...

3.7 A Pinch of Smiley

Percy.

Percy!

Percy?

I guess you're still asleep, little buddy. It's okay. I'm awake, I think. We'll talk later.

What's that sound? It's kind of a low sound. No, it's a mournful cry. Gee. Is that me?

As I opened my eyes as best I could, the first two people I saw were Richard and Mark. With their bright faces and adorable smiles, I just couldn't help but feel a pinch of smiley myself.

Why am I here? Where is here? Oh yeah. I had surgery and I'm in the hospital room. Oh, there's Richard and Mark. Ha, those smiles again.

"Hi, guys. How am I doing?"

"You're doing quite well, Jo-Ann. The surgery was not as long as they anticipated it would be. It lasted three hours and you spent some time in the recovery room. You're doing fine," said Mark.

"Nice to see you awake, Mom," said Richard.

"Sure nice to see both of my special fellas."

Percy?

Hmm ... No gurgle noises, no movement. My buddy must still be asleep, snuggled up in that little hammock.

What's that beeping? Gee. My thoughts are all over the place right now. Oh, it's me beeping. Gee. Look at all the machines around me. Pretty intimidating.

"Guys, are you sure I'm okay?"

"You're as okay as can be expected, Mom."

"My eyes are heavy. I think I'll take a little rest. See you guys later."

The lights are on in the room now, it must be dark outside. Oh great. I have an intravenous line in my arm. I hate those things. Can't seem to move my arm around. Where's my bedside table? I can't even see it, let alone reach it. Well, here we go again. Can't seem to move much, can't reach a thing, machines are still beeping, and I think I'm tied up in a knot. Oh, it's my hospital gown.

Percy! Earth to Percy. Come in Percy.

Still asleep, little buddy? Don't blame you.

Wow. The walls are really white, and oh, how smart, there's a whiteboard on the wall. There's writing on it but I just can't seem to focus my eyes to read it.

"Richard, what's written on the whiteboard?"

"Your nurse's name is written there. Your doctor's name, and some information about your medication."

"Oh, how smart is that. Very handy for the staff and for me. Well, handy for me when I'm able to read it. I actually don't feel my body very much right now. Is that a good sign?"

"Jo-Ann, your doctors have inserted an epidural in your spine, so painkilling drugs are passing into the small of your back via a tube, and they have you on other pain management drugs. I'm not surprised you can't feel your body, and that's what you need right now," said Mark.

"Oh, okay. You guys have been fantastic. Thank you for being with me today, but I think you've been through enough. Time to leave. Bye. See you tomorrow."

With kisses and very gentle embraces, my two special guys left, and I closed my eyes and drifted off into a strange sleep.

Meanwhile, when Mark arrived home — I'm sure very tired and relieved — he took the time to write and post an update on *The Ostomy Factor* blog to inform everyone of my day. Following is his posting:

Tuesday, March 19, 2013
After 3 hours of surgery, I am happy to report that Jo-Ann came through in great shape. The surgeon reports that all went better than expected. The peristomal hernia has been repaired, Percy is snuggled comfortably in his new sling. She is in great spirits and recovering very comfortably, (that is, the pain is being managed very well). As I left her at 8:30 PM, she was her old feisty self, joking with the nurses, and making a slew of

new friends on the hospital floor. She, I and Percy couldn't be more pleased (so far). Now the healing and recovery begins. More tomorrow.

3.8 Roommates

I opened my eyes and realized it was the morning, when, what to my wondering eyes should appear, but a blurred image of a man wearing a blue gown, standing near the foot of my bed, holding what looked like a wooden door.

"Hello," said the strange and rotund apparition.

"Hello," I responded, scarcely believing my eyes.

Gee. Is that an angel, another patient, and what is he doing holding a wooden door in his hands? Blinking my eyes a couple of times to try to focus them, while I checked in with my groggy brain, I opened my eyes wide again and sure enough, he was still standing there with a broad smile on his face.

"Hello," he said again.

"Oh hi, ah ... hem ... Why are you standing at the end of my bed?" I asked, still unsure if he was real or if he was a figment of my drugged mind.

"I'm waiting to go to the bathroom," he responded."The bathroom for our room is right here. Just past the end of your bed."

Oh great, I thought. I'm situated right on the path to the toilet facility in my room. The man in the blue gown then disappeared into the wall and a few moments later there was the sound of a flushing toilet. Okay. It's not the drugs, but what is a man doing in my room?

As it turns out, although we pay for a semi-private room, in most cases those rooms are already filled and we are then placed in a ward room. A ward room consists of four beds with patients and a bathroom. This time was the first time that the ward I was in was co-ed. My roommates consisted of two women and a man. Not sure how comfortable I feel about this, but it is what it is.

Percy?

There's no response to my calls to Percy. He's still asleep. No movement, no gurgles, no input nor output from him yet. Gosh, I miss my little buddy. Sure hope he wakes up soon, I need to get things moving or at the very least I will have to stay here longer. At the very most, I will become quite ill. Come on my little stoma, wake up, get on line.

"What's your name?" came the sound of a man's voice from the end of my bed.

"Jo-Ann."

"What you in for?"

"Um ... I've had abdominal surgery."

"How ya feeling?"

"Well, I'm really tired. I need to close my eyes and have a nap before my husband and my son arrive." I said this hoping he would get the message and respect my need for quiet.

"What's their names?"

"Mark and Richard."

"When they coming in?"

"I'm not sure, but I really need a bit of rest now."

"Oh sure, I'll just hop back in bed. See you later."

"Bye," I said with some relief.

"Don't you find the beds uncomfortable?" He asked from the other side of the curtain that was drawn between us.

Oh for goodness sake, I have a chatterbox as a ward mate. Great, I thought as I closed my eyes and fell into a fitful sleep. I did drift off, thanking my meds and my exhausted state, although I do remember hearing the man's voice drifting in and out of my consciousness. This was one of the times that I'm glad for my deaf left ear, with moderate hearing in my right ear only, and I did not have my hearing aids with me at hospital. Good grief!

Mark and Richard arrived and the man in the next bed introduced himself to them. In fact, he thought it was a good idea to be our entertainment co-ordinator. Even when the fellas closed the curtains around my bed for privacy, the man in blue continued to talk to us from his bed.

As the day rolled on, Mark stated that I needed some sleep and so could he refrain from trying to carry on a conversation with us. The man was a nice person, but we think he must have been very lonely and didn't seem to have any boundaries. The verbal chaos, clutter and confusion of sounds from him and his many trips to the bathroom continued for four more days. The day he left, we wished him well, and then I bathed in the blissful sounds of silence.

The Ostomy Factor blog — Mark's Posting
Wednesday March 20, 2013
Everything regarding Jo-Ann's recovery is going very well. She was able to go for short walks twice today. She is an extraordinary trooper and has the nurses charmed (big surprise). She is still eating clear liquids only, but hopefully that will change tomorrow. Percy is passing gas very frequently and making lots of noise (this is good since it means that he is progressing as well as Jo-Ann is). If the gas continues, she will progress to solid food (which will let Percy do his stuff ... do the thing he was born to do). Once all is working (Jo-Ann and Percy), they get to come home. More updates to follow. I have kept Jo-Ann posted regarding feedback. She sends her love and appreciates greatly hearing from you. It is much easier if we keep visitations in hospital to a minimum. I hope you understand. It is so that Jo-Ann can spend her energies getting ready to come home ... where you are welcome to visit anytime.

PART 4

Nerves and Nightmares

4.0 Gettin' the Job Done

Percy?

gurgle burble guggle

Oh dear, Percy. It all sounds like a bunch of babble to me. I don't think your little gut brain is in gear yet."

Be quiet, Jo-Ann!

Sorry Percy. I get it. I'm feeling pretty lousy too.

My day was very busy. It all started with the team of doctors who came by for a visit. A fine-looking group they were, even if it was only 7:00 a.m. They poked and prodded me as they examined my abdomen. Thanks to the pain management medication, I didn't feel much, only a slight bit of nausea. They discussed among themselves, and with a sunny bright smile on her face, my surgeon told me all was going as well as can be expected, and she would like me to continue taking short walks, and if the day goes well she was going to allow me to start solid food.

Wow. Wonderful. Terrific! Solid food tonight!

Hey, Percy. Did you hear that? Solid food. We're on our way!

I said, pleeeease be quiet, Jo-Ann."

Oh, Percy, don't be so grumpy. Wakey-wakey, little fella. You've got to get yourself ready. With solid food on the way, well, you need to be on top of your game.

I know Jo-Ann.

Next on my agenda is to pull myself together, get out of bed, and sit in the chair. I buzzed the nurse and in he came. Together, we made sure all of my lines to the machines keeping tabs on my vitals and the intravenous line (IV therapy in short) were in good order. I am a person who has had a life-long inclination for becoming tangled up in any string, thread, rope, hose, wire or what have you, within close proximity to me. Sure enough, even with the expert assistance of the nurse, I somehow got myself tangled and I got quite the tug on my intravenous line and a yank where it was inserted. Ouch!

With a few giggles and a couple more intricate moves, I finally became untangled and able to sit in the chair. Wow. What a struggle. It's taken me about three minutes to simply get out of bed, untangle, and then sit down. Ohhh, I'm dizzy. Sheesh, I'm whoozy. Wow. Beads of sweat are popping out all over my body. It's okay. I can do this.

"Hi." said the lady in the bed across from me.

"Hello."

"How are you feeling, young lady?"

"I'm doing okay, I guess. Took a lot to get out of bed, and I am not feeling the greatest right now."

"Yes dear, you look quite pale, but you'll feel better soon. Give it a bit of time."

"I will."

We began to have a lovely chitchat. She was elderly, 80 years plus I guesstimated. She was very gentle and very sweet. I sure am happy to have her as my roommate.

Then Mark arrived and he helped me back into bed. We enjoyed each other, and from time to time I would simply close my eyes and drift away, and this is when he brought out his book and quietly read while I was in my drug- and surgery-induced exhausted sleep.

Later in the afternoon, it was time to take a little walk. With my intravenous pole, bag and line at my side, we began to walk. Wow. My body is weak, my legs are wobbly, but I'm taking it one tiny step at a time. I'm so proud of myself.

Percy, look what we're doing!

Grumph, eeek!

Percy. Did you just blow a gassy gaffe? Sounded like you blew a raspberry.

I tried to contain my laughter so as not to burst open one of the staples that stretched from well above my belly button and down as low as can be.

We walked around and around the room, to the door of the room, and then we took a couple of steps out into the hall. My world was beginning to expand. Now back to bed with me. I'm exhausted.

At supper time, the staff brought a tray with a clear soup, crackers, weak tea, and Jell-O. I did not eat more than a couple of tablespoons of soup, had a sip of weak tea, and a spoonful of Jell-O. It wasn't much, but it was a start.

Between Mark and Richard, my day was wonderful.

After a final little walk, and when the fellas left, my lovely elderly roommate and I continued our delightful conversation. I did notice, as the minutes ticked by, that she seemed to become more and more weakened. I did not know what her medical situation was, but some time during the night she was moved out of the room. I never saw her again and found out the following day, she had passed away during the night.

I was quite sad but at the same time, I felt honoured that I'd had the opportunity to have met her, chitchat with her, and I feel I have been forever touched by her magnificence.

Good night, sweet lady, bon voyage, and thank you for you, I'll never forget you.

The Ostomy Factor blog — Mark's Posting
Thursday March 21, 2013
It was a good day today. Jo-Ann was able to get up and walk several times. The surgeon was able to allow her solid food as of 6 PM this evening thanks to Percy gettin' the job done. Pain management is going well, although because of the mesh inserted to repair the hernia, the surgeon indicated that there would be a higher level of pain during the healing process. Jo-Ann, as always, is insisting that the pain is nothing she can't handle, although I see her wince once in a while (which is unusual for her). All in all things are proceeding according to Hoyle. I am keeping her apprised regarding the many messages you have been sending. These are much appreciated. She sends you all her love. Stay tuned ...

4.1 Fighting the Raging Bull

Oh, yuk! I feel absolutely horrible. I think I'll place an ad advertising for a body double. They can take over for me in this bed so I can get out of this pain. Well, I know that won't work, but a girl can dream can't she? I'm so tired, I don't want to move, I don't want to think, I don't want to ... anything.

Percy. I haven't from heard you for a while now. You're just lying limp in your bag. Come on, little buddy. Percy. You need to be pooping, not pooped.

I guess I just have to face the reality of my life right now. I can hardly breath from the pain I'm feeling today, I'll try and sit in the chair for a while. What do I have to lose? Must say though, I sure don't feel like it today. I feel as though I'm falling and I have nowhere to go. I just want to lie here. In fact, I want to dry up and blow away in the breeze. There is no future I can see right now for myself, I just have this string of agonizing moments to get through.

The doctors have arrived. They seem to be somewhat concerned. Their sunny smiles have been replaced with serious gazes and they are speaking in quiet, almost inaudible, voices. Right now, I don't care. I just want to close my eyes and find a way to cut the demons out of my body and mind. Then, if I can, I want to lift my spirit so that I can fight this raging bull of pain and discomfort.

I'm tired. I'm going to sleep for a while, and I sure hope it's a long winter sleep. I need an escape. It's hard to watch myself break down. Right now I need to stay behind the metaphoric closed door. I'm keeping my emotions locked up inside of me. Thankfully, the wonderful nurses, Mark, and Richard seem to understand my need and efforts to tame the beast within.

I spent most of the day quite listless and I slept a lot. Thank goodness for blessed sleep. As the day passed, though, I started to feel a bit better. Not sure if the full body pain I had been experiencing all day had subsided but as the hours passed by, I was better able to tolerate the intensity.

I managed to get out of bed a number of times during the day and I sat in the chair for short periods of time. Although it felt like unsteady ground, I was able to take a few short walks. Hurrah for me. Well ... It sure didn't feel like a much of an hurrah but by late afternoon, although I still felt blue, I had now for the first time that day wanted to feel in the pink. Hmm ... That's a good sign.

The Ostomy Factor blog — Mark's Posting
Friday March 22, 2013
Oh well ... not a stellar day today. Unfortunately, pain management suffered a little ... not due to the outstanding care Jo-Ann is getting from hospital staff ... just due to the nature of the beast. The doctors warned us that pain levels might spike for a short while ... and spike they did. Jo-Ann had a bit of a rough morning and afternoon. Percy decided to take the day off (not terribly serious, but problematic) ... he needs to wake up soon and get back to doing what he does best. Late in the afternoon, the pain became more manageable. Jo-Ann's colour improved ... her energy came back ... but through it all she never lost her sense of humour or good spirits. Hopefully tomorrow will be a better day. When I left she was comfortable and eating a healthy supper.

4.2 Bolts of Lightning

Standing on the pillar of blood-red stone, the gun-metal black, indigo and grey clouds swirl and boil. Bolts of lightning crack and electrify my body and spirit. I stand strong against the wild wind and snapping whips of white fire that are striking my body, searing my skin with gashes that burn to the bone. The thunder is rumbling and exploding with deafening rage in my ears. The boiling and crashing water below is filled with unseen monsters. They are beckoning me to jump. I am bewitched by their seductive mystery. With all the power left in me, I lift my hand to the sky as I pull the bolts of lightning together to slay the monsters below and within. Without restraint, filled with anger and wild with emotion, I harness the power of the storm ...

"Oh, you startled me. Good morning. I was having an interesting dream," I said to the doctor standing by my bed.

"You had a rough night," she said.

"I feel like someone cut me in half and they've left all of the nerves in my body exposed to the wind, the rain, and all manner of harsh elements. I'm really feeling terrible"

"We know. I'm going to be sending you for a CTScan today. We're going to have a look and see what's happening inside. I'm also going to make a change to your pain management medication. It'll help you feel better. Do your best to relax. Take it easy. I'd like you to get out of bed and move, as well."

"Sure, I'll do my best," I said without much emotion nor energy.

It was a strange day for me. I spent most of it drifting off to sleep for long periods of time. When I did fall asleep, the wild dreams would come back. The good news in those dreams was the fact that, although I was being lured into the deep by unseen and seductive monsters, I was the hero who used all the tools around me to hold them at bay and eventually slay the monsters. I knew each time I woke up that I had many tools within me and others provided by modern medical science to beat back what was going wrong inside my body and my emotions. Each time, I was the heroine who won the day.

Wow. The subconscious is really amazing.

The Ostomy Factor blog — Mark's Posting
Saturday, March 23, 2013
A lousy day ... an as yet unknown complication has arisen. Jo-Ann had a terrible night (last night) ... awoken in the middle of it due to terrific pain. Doctor saw her this morning and took her off food and liquids ... back on the IV. She was sent down for a CTScan in the afternoon. We are still awaiting the results. They increased her pain medication which has helped somewhat ... but she hates the side effects (she gets a bit wonky). She was finally able to sleep heavily for about 45 minutes just before I left (which is good news). The pain was still at a high level when I left, but somewhat under control. All we can do now is wait. She is receiving terrific care (the staff has been terrific). Keep your fingers, toes, and eyes crossed. Percy is still being a bit stubborn ... not yet fully on the job. Hopefully we'll have good news from the doctor tomorrow.

4.3 Lost in My Sanity

Night is melting into day. Or is it day melting into night?

Percy, are you awake?

No response. Poor Percy is a tired and dragged out little stoma. Well, the rest of me feels that way, too. I thought by now I'd be feeling better. I'm so tired, so uncomfortable, I feel like someone has dragged me out to sea. I'm sinking.

Oh, I have an intravenous line hooked up again.

Hmm ... Sparks of lightning are flashing and slashing inside me. If the dreams could calm down, I might get a better sleep. Will do my best but it sure is getting tough.

"Hello, Jo-Ann." said the doctor with her team.

"Hi."

"It was a rough night. We're going to lay off the food for today and let your body rest. The test results have shown you have an infection and we're going to remove three of the staples at the bottom of the incision to allow the infection to drain."

"Sure, do what you have to do."

The staples were removed and I lay back and fell into a fitful sleep once again.

What a weird day. I can't figure out if it is day or night. Mark is here as he has been every day, sitting quietly reading his book. Must be day time.

"Honey, go home. I just need rest and I'm sure you need some time on your own, too. Go home, I'll be fine. I just need to sleep right now," I pleaded with him.

We kissed and he left.

I must have fallen asleep because when I opened my eyes, Mark was gone and there was a stranger at the end of my bed with a yellow sheet of paper that she was affixing to the bathroom door. Her blurred movements confused me. Was I dreaming again?

"Hello," I said.

"Oh! Hello. You startled me," said the now-rather-less-blurry image of a woman that turned and looked at me with a surprised look on her face.

"What are you doing?"

"I'm just putting this yellow paper on the door."

"A yellow paper. Isn't that interesting. Why are you doing that?"

"Oh, it's just a yellow paper. Nothing to be concerned about. But you can't use this bathroom.".

"Pardon me, but what's written on the yellow paper, and why can't I use that bathroom?"

"Nothing to worry about. Just don't use this bathroom," she said a little more forcefully.

"I'm not worried yet. I just want to know what the yellow paper is about and why I can't use the bathroom."

"I can't share the information with you. Just don't use this bathroom," she said with finality.

"Is the bathroom broken, or is it quarantined?" I once again attempted to understand what was happening.

"Take care now." She finished placing the yellow paper on the door, and she quickly left the room.

I know I'm not dreaming right now because I still see the irritating yellow paper on the bathroom door. I really want to know what it's about, and if I can't use the bathroom in my room, where is there another bathroom I can use? I've taken only a few steps out from my hospital room door and I haven't encountered any washrooms out there.

I buzzed for the nurse and the lovely young man appeared in front of me.

"There is a yellow paper on the bathroom door, and apparently I'm not to use the bathroom, what's that about?"

"Well, I'm not supposed to share the information. Just don't use the bathroom, and I'll go down the hall and get you a pamphlet."

Okay, I know I'm on a lot of drugs right now. I'm fixated on the silly yellow paper. I have been told enough times that I'm not to use the bathroom in my room and now a nurse is getting me a pamphlet. This is getting really bizarre.

A few moments later my nurse arrived with a pamphlet with the large letters "C-difficile" written at the top. Oh, dear. My thoughts went straight to a dear friend of mine who has a permanent ileostomy due to complications from *C. diff*. The butterflies started in my stomach, or I think it was butterflies, as I began to read.

The pamphlet stated that the average human digestive tract is home to as many as 1,000 species of microorganisms. Most of them are harmless — even helpful — under normal circumstances. But when something upsets the balance of these organisms in your gut, otherwise harmless bacteria can grow out of control and make you sick. One of the worst offenders is a bacterium called *Clostridium difficile*(*C. difficile*, also known as *C. diff*). As the bacteria overgrow, they release toxins that attack the lining of the intestines, causing a condition called *Clostridium difficile* colitis.

Oh, yuk. This is bad! Just then, the nurse returned to the room, wheeling a white commode. I watched him place the portable toilet into the middle of the room.

"Excuse me, everyone," he called out.

"For the time being, you'll not be able to use the bathroom in your room. You'll notice the yellow paper. This is a commode for your use."

Really, I thought. I don't know who in this room has or is suspected of having *C. difficile*, but if they don't want me to use the bathroom, I'm sure not sharing a commode with anyone!

The nurse quickly left the room at this point.

I continued to read the pamphlet. "relatively rare compared to other intestinal bacteria, *C. Diff* is one of the most important causes of infectious diarrhea."

Oh great. This is just getting better and better, I thought. Good news is, it's taken my mind off of my pain and discomfort. The bad news is, I'm frightened, anxious and I think I'm getting really worried for Percy and me.

"Symptoms of *C. difficile* infection can range from mild to life-threatening. Symptoms of mild cases include watery diarrhea, abdominal pain, loss of appetite, fever, and so on ..."

Oh, crap. I don't want to read any more of this pamphlet, I thought as my head bent forward and I continued to read more anyway.

"Symptoms of more severe cases include watery diarrhea, up to 15 times each day, severe abdominal pain, loss of appetite, fever, and so on ... some cases, *C. diff* infection can lead to a hole in the intestines, which can be fatal if not treated immediately. *C. diff* can be diagnosed by stool specimens tested for toxins. In some cases, a colonoscopy may be needed for diagnosis and more tests ordered."

Percy! You gotta wake up, little buddy. I really need you working now!

By this point I had read enough. I couldn't absorb any more information. I really need to sleep. I'm so exhausted. Don't know what tomorrow will bring. Hope we'll be okay. One thing for sure, I'm not sharing the commode with anyone. I want my own port-a-potty! I just feel so lost in my sanity and I don't have anything else to say!

The Ostomy Factor blog — Mark's Posting
Sunday, March 24, 2013
Wow ... what a relief today ... arrived at the hospital this AM and saw my cutie with a big smile on her face ... all rosy cheeked and everything. The problem had been a collection of seroma between the abdominal muscles and the skin. Seroma is a fluid that the body produces as a mechanism to fill any empty spaces left in the body after some surgeries. It is usually absorbed back into the body after healing commences. Unfortunately, while it collects it can augment pain. The medical staff had decided that since Jo-Ann was doing so well the first two days after surgery, they would wean her off of her pain medication sooner than planned. This reduction of pain medication plus the collection of seroma led to the perfect storm ... excruciating pain. The solution was to re-ramp up the pain medication. This provided the necessary relief to allow Jo-Ann to relax and sleep leading to the reduction and reabsorption of seroma fluid. Needless to say, we will continue the pain medication as long as required. Jo-Ann is many times better than she was yesterday ... the healing can resume. There was one blessing in this whole episode ... the CTScan results indicated that the surgery was completely successful ... everything was as it should be. Jo-Ann was amazing through

all this. *She was more worried about me and how I was doing (typical!). She sends her love to all of you and appreciates the messages, thoughts, and prayers. She actually apologized to me for giving us a scare. I left her this evening with a smile on her face looking forward to tomorrow.*

4.4 Wow, What A Relief

BRRT, PFFT, FLURPPPPPPP, Thwerrrpppp!

Percy, is that you?

Hi, Jo-Ann. Excuse me, lots of wind.

Oh, Percy. Welcome back!

Wow. Terrific. Happy, happy, skippy, skippy, little buddy.

I don't feel so good, Jo-Ann.

I know. I don't feel so good either, but this is shaping up to be a great day for us, little buddy.

Percy has indeed fully awakened and I just can't contain my joy. He's online, well not so strong yet, but online nonetheless. I even had a rather good sleep last night. I'm ready to climb upon the white commode and let nature take care of itself.

Hmm ... They didn't bring me my commode. It was at this time the nurse came into the room to check in on Percy and me.

"I notice you haven't had the opportunity to bring me my commode. I really need to go. I know you're busy, but could you bring it to me?"

"We don't have extra commodes. If you're not going to use the one provided in the room, there's a public washroom up the hall a bit, you can use."

Oh, well I need to expand my horizons, so it is up the hall with me. Goody. I get to see more of my world.

"Okay, but the problem is, I haven't ventured that far yet and I don't think I can make it on my own. And I need a lesson on how to get myself and my IV coordinated," I said.

"No worries, let me help you."

After a bit of manoeuvring and untangling myself from the plastic tubing, I moved slowly out of my room, heading for the hallway. I glanced at the irritating yellow sheet of paper on the bathroom door as I passed by. Into the world of a hospital hallway I hobbled. A world filled with people, sounds, and sparkling floors opened before me. I was thrilled and ready for the journey to my relief.

I was able to make it to the public bathroom. I broke out in a cold sweat and I felt very shaky. But I made it there and back to my room. Oh, it's great to be among the living again.

Upon my arrival back to my bed, in came the team of doctors for our daily consultation. They examined my still angry-red incision and complimented me on how much colour I had in my cheeks today.

"You're doing so much better today, we're removing the intravenous. You're going to eat some solid food, and we'll see how your day goes. If all goes well, we'd like to send you home possibly tomorrow or the next day. We feel you'll do well at home, probably better than here. We are arranging for Home Care to tend to the wound, and we're prescribing pain management medication," my oncologist/surgeon stated as I glanced at the yellow sheet of paper.

"That's terrific, I agree." I said.

"As you know, we'll be following up by telephone. You will have a follow-up appointment, and if there is anything you're concerned about, call the number we are providing you with, or come right in to hospital." She concluded our consultation with a gentle smile.

Percy. We're going home soon!

"FLURPPPPPPP, oh sorry. That's great, Jo-Ann!"

As the day progressed, although after the frequent and long-for-me trips to the public bathroom fatigued me, I felt better and better. Oh how wonderful I felt between my ears and relatively comfortable in my body.

The Ostomy Factor blog — Mark's Posting
Monday, March 25, 2013
Wow ... what a relief again today ... after the alleviation of the pain and stress, Percy came to life and is pooping away merrily

... doing the job he was born to do. Jo-Ann sends her love to all of you and appreciates the messages, thoughts, and prayers.

4.5 Home Sweet Home

"You had a good night last night?" asked the Doctor as she arrived in the room with one of her residents.

"Yes. Percy and I had a great night last night. We're hoping that you'll allow us to go home today. Is that possible?" I sat up as straight and perky as I possibly could manage.

"I think that's a good idea. We've made the Home Care arrangements, I have your prescriptions ready, so, as soon as Mark arrives, you are good to go."

Yippee ki yay, Percy. It's home sweet home for us.

I'm ready, Jo-Ann.

Mark could not come soon enough for Percy and me. When he arrived, he packed up our case with my few toiletries and Percy's equipment. He loaded us into the wheelchair, and we said our goodbyes to the staff of the Ottawa Hospital who had been so wonderful, attentive, and professionally sympathetic to Percy, Mark and me. Goodbye and thank you to all.

As we exited through the sliding door and into the sunshine, I drank in as much of the fresh air as I could. It is great to be alive!

The Ostomy Factor blog — Mark's Posting
Tuesday, March 26, 2013
Jo-Ann and Percy are home ... I am content!

PART 5

Emergence

5.0 Percy Loves Bling

When I arrived home, my little cat Niki was so excited to see me, she jumped on the bed and began to rub her head on my arm.

"Hi, Niki. Yep, we're home and this time, to stay. Glad to see you, too."

Ding dong went the door bell, Richard has arrived and he headed upstairs and to sit on the bed with Niki, Percy and me while Mark went out to the pharmacy to fill the prescriptions. Wow. I'm really home.

Ding dong. This time, large boxes of wound care supplies arrived and were delivered to my bedroom. Just as it had been during recovery from the July 21, 2011 surgery, the bedroom once again was quickly becoming a pharmaceutical dispensary.

Ding dong went the doorbell again. This time it was the Home Care nurse. Both Mark and Richard greeted her and led her upstairs to my bed where I was holding court. This delightful lady introduced herself with a big smile and indicated to me she would be visiting me every day for as long as she was needed for my wound care. She explained that she would be caring for my 7-inch abdominal wound. Due to the fact that three staples had to be removed due to infection, she was also required to pack the wound so it would heal from the inside out. As she worked with the incision area, and in particular the open wound, I noticed an interesting silvery-looking packing she was inserting into the wound.

"Wow, that's fancy looking packing."

"It's actually silver. Silver has been used in treating wounds for some time. Silver has an array of beneficial effects in promoting healing. Basically, silver maintains tissue hydration while controlling bacteria. In fact, silver has been recognized for centuries as a useful antimicrobial agent. You know, in the early nineteenth century, surgeons used silver sutures to close incisions in some surgeries. You don't have an allergy to metal do you?"

"No, I don't. I love silver. Look, Percy, you're surrounded with bling." I giggled.

At this point, she looked around to introduce herself to the Percy fella. She looked at Mark, then Richard, then scanned the room, then looked back at me with a questioning look on her face.

"Oh, Percy is not a person, Percy is my stoma." I said.

"I've heard of some people naming their stoma. Well, hello, Percy. I'm going to be taking very good care of you."

When she left, I felt a big wave of fatigue come over me. It was a good day and an exciting day, but I felt spent and it was time for a nap.

When I awakened a while later, I noticed Mark and Richard reviewing the documents from the hospital that were sent home with me. They lined up the many medications. They began setting up my medication schedule. As I lay in bed, feeling quite incapable of doing anything for myself, I was once again amazed by my two caregivers.

Some nerves in my abdomen were waking up reminding us it was time to take some pain management medication.

Time to drift off but before I do, I just want to say thank you, thank you that I made it through the surgery, I don't have *C. diff*, and I can return to the business of my spectacular recovery.

5.1 We're Back

Hey, Percy.

Yes, Jo-Ann.

How are you feeling?

Poopy, figuratively. Not really, literally, yet!

Yes, I know, little buddy. The good news is an enterostomal therapy nurse (ET Nurse) will be visiting us today. You've really had a time of it, Percy. You were re-seated, and this caused you a great deal of trauma.

Tell me about it, I'm swollen, flush with fever, and I'm not fully online yet. I haven't been able to produce a decent poop for us for nine days now. Sheesh!

Okay, Mr. Grumpy Pouch, I'm taking stool softeners in the hopes that will help you. I think you're simply traumatized by the whole situation.

Let's change the subject, Jo-Ann.

Yes. It's better if I can take my mind off illness so that I can get on with our spectacular recovery, again ... still ...

Percy and I are very grateful for the many folks we know and those we don't know personally for all of their support and love. As Mark read the many blog comments, cards, and email messages from so many, I sure feel we're together on this interesting journey.

I'm now able to sit for short periods of time at the computer. I'm very excited that I've been able to get back to writing my blog publications. I have made it a point to publish one blog per month, and I'm so glad I haven't missed a month yet. Unfortunately, I'm still on morphine and other pain management medications, so I'm being extra careful writing and hoping that my blog posts make sense. If not, I can always blame it on the meds.

Considering what has occurred in the past few weeks, I really feel I'm doing as well as possible. I have a Home Care nurse that comes in each day to attend to my wound care. Unfortunately, I have had to endure a number of complications that will be cleared up soon. I contracted a bladder infection, and an infection in the wound while in hospital. Some more of the staples have had to be removed, and so, I have deep holes in the area of the incision that must heal from deep inside and then out to the surface of my skin.

I have been put on antibiotics, and now I'm enjoying a full-blown case of thrush. Oh, the fun never ends. At least I'm not dealing with *C. difficile*. Must say, I've referred to my trusty pamphlet so many times now that it's getting ratty looking.

My spirits are high and unlike Percy, I'm not Ms. Grumpy Pants yet. Hope I can keep this up. Percy and my body is another story entirely and I am waiting for the days when I can say, "Hmm ... I'm feeling better with each passing day.

5.2 Thar She Blows

The healing journey is an interesting dance. It's one step at a time forward with a leap or a bound thrown in for good measure. Then there's the sideways stomp and the occasional backslide. Yet progress is made in this freestyle dance.

Percy continues to have a challenging time of it. Little Percy pooper is pooped out for the time being. The good news is, he is slowly but surely waking up and we're anticipating Percy will return to his healthy pungent self and once again will be immersing himself in his liquidation business. What a trooper.

I continue to make the necessary healing strides with the help of Mark, the Home Care nurses, and my cheerleading friends and family. They have joined me in the healing dance and I am grateful for them. I continue to ingest a cocktail of pain management drugs that are really making my brain wonky, I'm on two antibiotic prescriptions at this time and I have a few more prescriptions thrown in for good measure.

Mentioning pain management drugs and their affects, Percy informed me he was looking forward to posting the next blog. Not sure what he'll come up with, but I'm expecting now that he seems to be feeling a bit better that I'll be at the butt end of his potty humour. Should be interesting.

The days flowed one into the other and on Wednesday, April 3, I realized there were only 24 hours left and the Home Care nurse would be removing the remaining twenty-one of the original thirty-one surgical staples. Now I'm not normally a Nervous Nellie, but in my rather-more-distant past, when surgical stitches had been removed, the whole incision opened up and came fully apart. A traumatic experience, to say the least.

And so, the whole night before, "Thar She Blows" screamed throughout my dream-filled night. I woke up in the morning with the terrible image still in my mind as I awaited my Home Care nurse's arrival. I had informed her of my concerns the day before, so when she arrived, she was aware of my anxiety and was extremely considerate.

She settled into her task and one by one removed the staples. I'm glad to say it all went exceedingly well. The incision did not open up and there was no Thar She Blows. Must say, I'm really relieved this stage of the healing journey is behind me, and I'm looking forward to the day when I'm well enough to dream "Thar She Goes."

5.3 Percy's Bedtime Story

Our healing journey is filled with days that present Percy and me with challenges and with triumphs. One of the frustrating aspects since the surgery, is my difficulty in finding a pain-free sleeping position as I wean myself off the pain-management medication. This has been rather disconcerting to say the least.

Jo-Ann.

Yes, Percy.

Can I share some of your thoughts in this chapter?

What thoughts are you referring to, Percy?

Um ... Well ... The ones that you have about how you don't stay frustrated for too long.

Sure, you can share those thoughts.

Ahem. As Jo-Ann mentioned, she is weaning herself off the pain-management medication. This has been rather disconcerting. Never ones to be in a state of frustration for too long, Jo-Ann and I are facing the challenge by reaching into our bag of tricks — bags are my specialty — and coming up with a resourceful solution.

Ongoing since I was created, Jo-Ann has, from time to time, had difficulty staying asleep all night. We're incontinent, so there are nights when I'm active and we have to do our maintenance. No matter what time it is, it's not always easy to go right back to sleep.

No use tossing, turning, getting frustrated or fretting, because sometimes we meditate, we pray, we count sheep, we talk to long-dead friends and relatives, and so on. These don't work every time, though. Jo-Ann isn't always sure when I'm finished my activities. I've decided these nights are not so bad really and that's because Jo-Ann and I will tell a bedtime story. She fills her head with images and stretches her imagination. Her stories are usually quite funny and they have a moral to each and every one of them. In the quiet of the night, when everyone is asleep, together we weave the fabric of our imaginations and we walk through the misty night tracts, to arrive at the Runs River in the land of Flange. On some of our visits, we dance with Prince Colon. On other nights, we join Lady Catheter of Tube for some titillating conversations.

So if you have one of those nights ... You know, the ones where you just have to go with the flow? Here's one of our bedtime stories to entertain you and help you fall asleep.

The Duke Of Flange

Long ago there lived the Duke of Flange who was responsible for overseeing the Department of Incontinence Difficulties. Every day, the Duke would say, "If only we could control the flow of the Runs River." For a long time there was no control.

Then there came the day of the great Esprit de Corps Festival. The harvest was in and many came from all over to feast and celebrate. As each attempted to cross the Runs River, the raging torrent bubbled and boiled making the crossing treacherous indeed. To the dismay of the Duke of Flange, most were turning back. It was not safe.

The Duke quickly called together the Privy Council to once and for all find a way to control the Runs River. Sir Paper of Toilet, Lady Irritable of Bowel, Prince Colon, Queen Urethra and King Convexity were the first to arrive, followed by many others. They discussed, considered and discussed the matter some more, but no solutions came to mind. Then, in their darkest moments of dismay, someone quietly entered.

"My name is Percy. I am but a humble stoma. We have long awaited our Festival and for our invited guests to arrive." He smiled. "I have the solution." Everyone went silent and turned to hear what the humble stoma had to say.

"The Runs River has a mighty flow. This flow reminds us of the nutrients of the land that we need in order to stay healthy and prosperous. There are no blockages. As the River twists through the narrows, it provides us with all that is good. Let us not block the movement. Let us not stem the flow. Instead, let us wait it out. Have patience. The Runs River does not always flow so wild. After the time of the great torrent, the Runs River always returns to normal. It is then that we will send out the messengers and invite all to join in our Festival, and we will feast as we celebrate."

Everyone was silent, no sound was made. It was then that the Duke of Flange embraced and encircled Percy, the humble stoma, and shouted, "Your words are wise. We will wait out the great torrent, and then all will be well."

King Convexity and Queen Urethra stepped forward and declared, "From this day forward, you will be addressed as and will hold the title: Stoma, Eol of Poopology. Thank you for your great service."

Everyone cheered.

I do hope you enjoyed one of our bedtime story adventures, the moral of this story is: We can't control everything but we can take control. We are incontinent. That is our challenge. Humour, creativity and some resourcefulness is our victory.

Thank you for making me the hero of the story. Jo-Ann. I'm touched.

You're welcome, Percy. Let's face it, you are the hero of my life story, for without you, there is no me. Remember, though, stay humble, my little stoma, stay humble.

5.4 Percy Sees Stars

It's hard for me to be humble when you look back on my history, Jo-Ann.

Here we go. Yes, Percy. You're a pretty amazing stoma. But I must say, all stomas are amazing.

I suppose so, Jo-Ann.

Okay, Percy. Let's take a look back at what you've done in the past couple of years.

During our recovery, Percy, as in the past, has become the star of the show. Or maybe he's just seeing stars?

Hey.

Sorry, Percy. I couldn't resist.

Proceed, Jo-Ann.

Let's step back and find out how all this came about.

Percy Stoma's Biography

Created in Ottawa, Canada on the 21st of July, 2011, Percy started his existence by being a life saver, right from the get-go. His first of many public presentations was to the resident ET nurse, within a few days of creation at the Ottawa Hospital. He returned to Orleans, Ontario later that month and with an un-snap of his bag, he continued to perform presentations for a multitude of audiences that included community ET nurses, Home Care nurses, and doctors, who, in his opinion, made him an overnight success.

Percy settled down to the life of a stoma, pooping, passing wind, writing and posting blogs while at the same time broadening his activities as a model for custom-designed haute pooture underwear that accommodate stomas and their bags, while providing abdominal support.

Percy's reputation grew steadily, helped by his earning of an EoL of Poopology (EoL, Experience of Life), given to him to celebrate Jo-Ann's recovery from a major illness by providing her with a second chance at life.

During 2012, Percy saw continued recovery and the publication of a book based on his creation, his life and his adventures. He was asked to be the model for an oil painting titled "Percy, a Self-Portrait" that graces the front cover of *Better WITH a Bag than IN a Bag.*

More public presentations have followed as he was uplifted by a honey-dew-melon-sized parastomal hernia. These included nurses, ET nurses, specialists, and physicians. A second collaboration with the surgeon who had originally created him, resulted in major surgery in March of 2013, a surgery performed with the intent of designing an internal environment conducive for a higher quality of life for Percy.

Percy has now re-united with Home Care nurses on a daily basis for wound care, has visited the hospital emergency for a post-surgery concern, and was recently measured and fitted for a customized abdominal hernia belt. (For more information on hernia belts go to the "Information, Hints & Tips" section.) His most ambitious work is yet come, a full recovery without a parastomal hernia re-occurrence.

Now I must admit that Percy has been enduringly popular as we remove his bag and he bares himself without being self-conscious during his private and public medical presentations. He is quite proud of his new and more svelte profile, much to my discomfort and embarrassment due to my desire for privacy.

Percy not withstanding, most of us feel our dignity is compromised when, due to medical issues, we are required to expose and share our body and/or parts of it that we would much rather keep private. Understandable and normal, I feel. embarrassment aside, no matter the body or life part that is potentially ill, injured, or in recovery, we should have regular check-ups. It's important that we indulge in medical presentations and scrutiny. The jury is still out as to whether Percy is the star of the show or he's just seeing stars. I regard his performances as private and public presentations that are an advantage to both of us. What I'm saying here is, next time you have to bare and share a part of yourself that you would rather not make public (like a colonoscopy for example), just think of it as a command performance from which you will benefit; and know you will be glad that you attended, even if it strikes an emotional chord.

You ate some cabbage today, Jo-Ann. Maybe I am just seeing stars.

5.5 One of the Greatest Gifts

Woo hoo, skippy, skippy, and resounding cheer from Percy. It's Thursday, May 2, 2013, and Percy and I have reached a milestone. Our Home Care nurse has signed us off today. For the past six weeks she has visited us once a day, then every second day, and finally in the past two weeks, every third day, all the while gently tending to my surgery wound care. She always arrived with a smile, a big hello, and then settled down to inspect the wound and administer her healing magic. Always the professional with that personal touch.

Now as Percy has remarked to me on more than a few occasions this past week, "Poopologically speaking, we should be ecstatic." Yet I find myself feeling strangely adrift. I have taken the last couple of days to explore this odd feeling and have come to a realization:

When we are vulnerable, injured, in pain, and require expertise beyond ourselves, we place a great deal of confidence in those folks who are there to help us. They are in our lives during our time of weakness, and we look forward to their being there with us. We trust they have the know-how to keep us safe as they encourage us along our healing journey. They are our cheerleaders standing behind and with us along the way. Then the day comes when we don't need them anymore. This bond we had established, this healing team that scored so many goals, is now disbanded ...

Of course, it is time to move on. The healing is underway and full recovery is the ultimate goal. As humans, we need to live with, for, and by one another. So thank you to all of the health care professionals for your healing magic and for being the best cheerleaders a patient could hope for.

My musings have brought me to other members of the healing team: my personal caregiver, Mark, and my family. I'm so fortunate to have people who care. Reminiscing about the past few years, I see that I endured my illness, near death, two major surgeries, recovery that has now taken up years of my life, and through it all, we were together, we were and are a team, and we fought the good fight. I encourage everyone to think about helping others in their time of need if for no other reason than you just never know when you may need that shoulder to lean on. Your love, care and commitment is one of the greatest gifts you will ever give.

PART 6

Celebration

6.0 Wisdom and Living Examples

So much to look forward to, so much spectacular healing to achieve, and now it is time for getting on with, getting on with.

Jo-Ann, let's take an inventory again.

Good idea, Percy.

Challenge list:

I poop in a bag (well that's a given and for the rest of my life)

I'm still having to self-catheterize

I have drop foot

I have medication-induced psoriasis (not so much on hands now, still on heels and bottom of feet)

I must continue my post-surgery body, mind and spirit recovery

Wow. We've eliminated:

Parastomal hernia (this is huge! Percy and the rest of my colon are not in danger of strangulation any longer)

I am free of pre-surgery nervous jitters and preparation

Two down and three more to eliminate. We're on our way to that spectacular recovery we've been working so hard to achieve, Percy.

Terrific, Jo-Ann! Where do we go from here?

Good question, Percy.

I strongly trust in a mind/body connection. During the worst of times, this attitude and approach uplifted me and carried me over the abyss where I could have easily let go, let myself fall, and cease to exist. I do believe my mind and emotions have played a critical role in my health. Hippocrates, the father of Western medicine, taught there is an interconnection between mind and body in healing when he emphasized that good health depends on a balance of mind, body, and environment.

This understanding was permanently planted into my mindset by two amazing women, my Granny and my Mom.

Quite few years ago, when I was in my early teenage years, Granny suffered a stroke. The left side of her body was affected, initially causing her to be unable to move her arm, hand and fingers. On the day before her birthday, my Auntie, her eldest daughter, visited her in hospital. Granny mentioned that it was Auntie's birthday the following day but, of course, Granny did not have a gift for her.

In response, Auntie told to her, "Oh that's okay, the best gift you can give me is to get well. That's the only present I want."

The following day, Auntie arrived to celebrate her birthday with Granny. When Auntie exited the elevator at the hospital, a nurse gave her one of those knowing smiles, a smile that made her suspect the nurse knew something Auntie didn't. When she entered the room Granny was sitting up and looking fresh and pretty, and it was at this time she said, "I have your birthday present."

Auntie said, "Oh that's lovely," as she wondered and waited. It was at this time that Granny lifted her arm up from the bed, crossed it over her lap, and then returned it to her side again. Amazing! The day before, Granny could not achieve this, and this day, she had given this profound gift all under her own power. This movement was her gift to her daughter.

Auntie was extremely delighted as a nurse entered the room stating, "Your Mom worked all night to lift her arm. She didn't give up. She focused, concentrated, and she has been successful!"

In time, Granny went on to stand, walk, and move her arm and hands again. Her fingers did not fully come back to the full dexterity as they had been before the stroke, though. I remember her habit of placing a tea towel in her left hand and squeezing it shut on the towel with her right hand, and then, with tea towel in hand being as useful as possible, she went about her business of working in the kitchen.

She amazed me and reinforced the concept that even when the odds can be stacked against you, your mindset is a valuable tool for achieving goals that you set out for yourself, goals that in the beginning can seem less than possible.

The second incident that finally ingrained the mind/body connection into my belief system occurred when I was in my late teens. It was December 1, 1973 and a cold winter day when Mom and Dad were travelling home from a shopping trip in Barrie, Ontario. They were on their way back to our home at Canadian Forces Base Borden. Mom was driving the car and Dad was in the passenger seat, the car was filled with groceries, and two sets of cross-country skis and ski poles, all stowed away in the back seat area.

Bridges will freeze before a road surface will. Due to freezing wind striking the bridge above and below, a bridge will lose heat from every side. The road is only losing heat from its surface. Even while the temperature on the road surface is dropping, the heat underneath the road keeps it warm enough to prevent icing as temperatures in the atmosphere drop below freezing. Bridges have no way of trapping any heat so they will continually lose heat and freeze shortly after temperatures in the atmosphere are at the freezing point. As a result, a bridge will follow the air temperature very closely. If the air temperature falls below freezing, a bridge's surface will fall below freezing very quickly. Rain or snow, therefore, will freeze and stick to the bridge before the road will be icy.

This is what happened on that fateful day. As the car traversed the bridge, control was lost due to the icy surface. Slipping and sliding across the bridge, the car skidded off just where the bridge ended and the road surface began. It flipped end over end, throwing Mom 18 meters (approximately 60 feet) onto the embankment of the Nottawasaga River. Dad remained in the car that eventually hung itself upside down on a farmer's fence.

Mom sustained compound pelvic fractures, a broken hip, and head injuries. Doctors advised she should be placed in a body cast for at least nine months. As it turned out, she was not put in a body cast and I do think Mom had something to do with this decision. But as one can imagine, she was to remain in hospital for a lengthy period of time. The physicians felt it would be a long recovery, and there would be long-term home care required while she healed and recovered as much as her body possibly could.

As Christmas approached, Mom's body was still very broken and the doctors prepared her for their reality that she would be spending Christmas in hospital. Well! Mom would have none of that! She emphatically told us that she would be well enough to be released from hospital by Christmas Day, there was no way her family would be spending that special day in hospital as she intended to celebrate at home with her family.

We humoured her, all the while planning on how we could make her hospital room as Christmassy as possible, and designing the best Christmas Day celebration in hospital as we could. As mentioned, Mom had other plans, and so, two days before Christmas, Mom had made such progress that the doctors agreed she could leave hospital and continue her recovery at home as an outpatient. At home, we circled the wagons around her and we were delighted to be together in our own home, and able to celebrate the special day with Mom holding court as she lay in repose. We decorated the tree, listened to Christmas music, laughed and celebrated the fact that we were once again together as a family.

As it was, I had been scheduled to become married in April, 1974. Mom would probably not be able to endure a full day as the mother-of-the-bride let alone be able to walk well yet, so I suggested we postpone the wedding. Mom would have nothing to do with this and said the wedding would happen as planned. She was determined that she would be ready. December moved into January and February and Mom continued to recover. As the winter began to melt away, Mom was now able to walk around for short distances with a cane. Considering, according to the doctor's plan, that she would still have been in a body cast, here she was involved in the many activities leading up to the wedding of her daughter.

The big day arrived and it was the morning of my wedding day. The house was filled with friends and family, the homemade soup was bubbling on the stove and glorious merriment permeated throughout. It was at this time that Mom quietly came into my room with her cane in hand. She tenderly touched me on the shoulder, wished me love, then lifted her cane, hung it up in my closet and said, "See this cane? I'm finished with it. I'm not going to need to use it again. This is my little gift for you today."

With tears of joy in my eyes, and concern that Mom was going to go through a whole wedding day without the support of her cane, I was amazed once and again by her, by her strength of mind, emotions and body that brought her to the point that within four months she was able to hang up her cane and step out in life whole and determined to get on with her life.

Through Granny and Mom's teachings, it was time to set my mind, body and emotions in motion and get on with getting on. Thank you, my amazing and strong matriarchs, for your wisdom and living example of what a person — even an ordinary person such as I — can accomplish if I put my mind to it.

6.1 Catching on like a House on Fire

Granny and Mom achieved seemingly spectacular and magical recoveries, not through sitting and waiting for time to heal them. Instead, they set recovery/healing goals, focused, applied determination, hard work and imagination, and believed they could realize as much of what is as humanly possible.

Albert Einstein was a German-born theoretical physicist. His work is also known for its influence on the philosophy of science. He developed the General Theory of Relativity, one of the two pillars of modern physics (alongside quantum mechanics). Einstein is best known in popular culture for his mass-energy equivalence formula $E=mc^2$ (which has been dubbed "the world's most famous equation"). Another of Einstein's quotes is one I am seriously affected by:

"Imagination is more important than knowledge. For knowledge is limited to all we now know and understand, while imagination embraces the entire world and all there ever will be to know and understand." This singularly powerful message opens my mind and emotional heart to the potential for physical possibilities without any borders.

From the day I was informed I had drop foot, I embarked on a visualization project for myself. Visualization for me is the act of recalling or forming mental images/pictures that are perceptible to my mind and imagination. It is a perception practice I have worked with for many years of my life with the purpose and the expectation of affecting my inner and outer world. When I found out about the drop foot, I immediately started envisioning a radiant tree with branches that glowed, brilliant leaves reaching out, and luminous roots surging and growing with lustrous energy. As I set my focus on this vision in a mind free of judgement and without any encumbrance, my intent was to heal the nerves of my body. I'm visualizing for my nerves so that my mind will know and assist them to awaken, build new neurological bridges, connect, and transmit proper signals. It is due to nerve damage from the original disease and invasive surgery required that I have drop foot, and I am required to self-catheterize. In addition, healthy transmitting nerves are an asset to post-surgery body recovery.

(The job of the nerves is to transmit signals that the brain sends out to the rest of the body in order to tell it what to do. Every time we perform an action, our brain will tell a specific part of our body exactly how to move in order to accomplish that task, and this message is transmitted very quickly through our nerves.)

Looking at the life journey I have experienced during the past ten months during my recovery and then undergoing major surgery once again, I found myself immersed in the grieving process. Throughout the process, I have been repeatedly reminded that there are so many changes that occur for anyone and everyone when they must face illness, a significant emotional event, or life alteration(s), whether chosen or thrust upon them. The grieving process is described as stages, although, as we know, we will experience the stages not necessarily one after the other; instead, we feel any one of them at any given time and sometimes, we feel all of them at the same time. As I progressed through the stages of shock, denial, bargaining, anger, depression ...

Excuse me, Jo-Ann.

Yes, little buddy.

We've arrived at Acceptance. *Am I on the right track here?*

We're both on the right track now, little buddy!

Inspired by Granny and Mom, their zest for life is music to my heart, their wisdom, nourishment for my mind that is always high-octane fuel for my imagination which is now in full gear, and so, it is time to move forward with enthusiasm and personal power. We're making a pivotal step here.

I have been off of the pain medication for over a month and it is time to get behind the wheel of the car and feel freedom again and expand my horizons. Chris and Beth's wedding is next month and I think I'll try on the dress I purchased in Florida. I've lost weight, and although I'm still a bit swollen, the original melon-sized lump under Percy is shrinking by the day. Sure do hope I can feel good wearing our dress.

Percy!

Yesssss.

The dress fits. It looks really nice. I'm so happy.

Yup. It feels good for me, too.

The month of June seemed to fly by as we prepared for the big event that would take place at Manora Park Pavilion, Mono, Ontario.

Percy?

Yessss, again.

I may be mistaken, but I seem to feel sensations when I have to pee.

Really? Wow. That's terrific!

It was true. As each day in the month of June came and went, I could feel the sensation of a full bladder and when I needed to void. After some checking and experimentation, I am indeed now in full control of voiding. That amazing visualized tree is doing its magic!

I can now remove self-catheterization from my challenge list. Three down and two to go. With a dollop of hope for good measure, I continue to focus on psoriasis management, all the while giving diligent attention to the rhythm of my post-surgery body, mind and spirit recovery.

It's now two weeks to the wedding celebration and I'm actually noticing that my left foot seems to be more in step with my right foot. Could it be that the nerves in my lower spine are also coming back on line? I'll give it a little more time before I risk jumping with joy.

Jo-Ann, your glowing tree is catching on like a house on fire!

It sure seems to be, Percy. Wow. We have so much to look forward to.

6.2 Best Friends Forever

I'm excited and a bit nervous, Percy.

Oh, dear. You know that can be a bit of trouble for me.

Yes, I know. I'm doing my best to stay balanced.

I'm excited because I really think Beth and Chris are a perfect passionate match, and I'm so happy for them. I'm also excited because after the wedding weekend, we have decided to visit my friend Lynn, whom I met forty years ago. I'm nervous because this is the first long drive we're taking since the surgery in March. I hope Percy and I can physically handle it. From our home to Mono, Ontario is 483 kilometres (approximately 300 miles) about a five and a half-hour drive with stops; then from there to my friend Lynn's home is another 149 kilometres (approximately 93 miles).

My friendship with Lynn is an interesting experience for both of us. I met Lynn when I moved from Nova Scotia to Ontario in 1962, to Canadian Forces Base Borden, Ontario. This was a particularly emotional move for me as I was 16 years old, and being a teenager, I had an established social group in Nova Scotia, and this is very important for a teen. Prior to the move to CFB Borden, I had spent ten years of my life living by the ocean, which I took full advantage of. I played in the ocean, I explored tidal pools, I marvelled at the changing moods and colours of the ocean. I had earned my Third Standard in Seamanship with Maritime Command and with the wind in my sails and me at the helm, I had sailed beautiful Halifax harbour with its miles of shoreline and its graceful lighthouse. I had made wonderful friends through a camping club our family belonged to, friends who had found their way into my heart and have remained there to this day. All of a sudden in the midst of my teenage angst, I was being uprooted, ripped from the ground I had adopted and loved, and I had to move to a place that was not graced with the ocean, and where I didn't know anyone. It would prove to be an intense experience that summer, to say the least.

Arriving at CFB Borden with no friend to call, no boat to sail, no ocean shore to explore and no ocean breeze to clear my mind, I felt lost. About a week into my homesickness and despair, I met a girl walking down the street. She smiled and gave me a big hello. Wow. She had actually taken the time to stop and greet a perfect stranger. She had a beautiful smile and I liked her immediately. She told me her name was Lynn and pointed out where she lived. As it turned out, she lived about four houses down from me. I had a glimmer of hope that there were nice people in this place, and I could possibly make a good friend to her.

For five days I sat out on our front lawn in the hopes Lynn would walk down the street again. She did, and when I saw her, I jumped up and ran to her to say hello. She gave me an ear to ear smile and asked if I would like to come to her house and hang out. I was ecstatic. She wanted to be my friend!

I did go to her house, met her family, and spent the rest of the summer hanging out with her, playing with her and her siblings, and blending in with her family. It was a glorious summer, after all, although I truly missed the ocean and my only sibling Diane who had stayed back in Nova Scotia to work her summer job.

At the end of August, before school began, Lynn told me she and her family were moving. I can't tell you how devastated I was to hear this. She was my friend, her family was my adopted family, we were friend-sisters and I just knew I would never forget her. She did move away at the end of summer, and I started my new school not knowing anyone, and as young people are, we lost touch with one another.

I missed her then, and never stopped missing her throughout my life. Although I did not know what had happened to her through the years, I always thought of her, and in my heart and mind I wished her the best in the hopes that her life would turn out the way she wanted it to. There were so many hopes and dreams that we had shared during that glorious summer that seemed to last forever, and then was gone in the blink of an eye.

As life will have it, a short while ago, my sister, Diane, had called me and stated that she had just come upon a website that announced the Base Borden Collegiate High School Reunion site that stated it had been a success. We were both disappointed that we had not known a reunion happened, although it turns out I would not have been able to attend as I was in recovery. With her on her computer at her home and with me on my computer at my home, and connected by phone, we explored the site together. There were many names we recognized although the faces had changed in the forty years that had lapsed since we were in high school. It was a true delight travelling down memory lane for both Diane and me.

A few days later, Diane emailed me stating that she had left her name and email address on the Base Borden School Reunion website in the hopes that someone from her past would contact her. She did indeed receive an email but it was not for her.

It read: name is Lynn, I believe you have a sister with the name Jo-Ann. If so could you forward my email address to her. If you're not her sister, then thank you and I'm sorry to have disturbed you.

I did not recognize the last name given in the email so did not know who this person was, but I did respond. Well! What to my surprise when I realized that Lynn was actually my dear friend from that glorious sweet-16 summer. I was delighted, excited and truly amazed that life had given my dear friend back to me after all these years.

She, too, had never forgotten me and stated that she had always considered me her best childhood friend even though, as we realized, we had only known each other in Borden less than three months. As it turns out, we both shared the same sentiments for each other then and this many years later. We have reconnected on all levels, although she lives about a seven-hour drive west of us. Living in the age of communication today has ensured that we will never lose each other again. With the wedding five hours west of us, it will be a short hop, skip and a jump to Lynn's home. I can't wait to see her, share with her, and introduce Mark and Percy to her.

True friendship is something noble and great. The company of friends adds to our happiness and makes life interesting. A true friend understands us and appreciates our circumstances and our problems. A true friend shares our joys and misfortunes. I have certainly had the pleasure to be on the receiving end of friendship throughout my illness and surgeries of the past few years. I have appreciated every phone call, get well soon card, and delicious food our friends and family took the time and effort to share with Mark, Percy and me.

And so, Mark, Percy, and I are getting ready to embark on our first road trip since the surgery in March, to celebrate the joining of daughter Beth and her best friend Chris in matrimony, and then to celebrate and rejoin with my best friend from long ago.

6.3 Special Moments with Special People

Percy's new dress is carefully packed. Percy's ostomy equipment has been inventoried and is now packed as well. It's time to head out for another adventure. Beth, Chris, and Lynn, here we come!

Percy, you're really quiet. Are you okay?

Oh yes, I'm just relaxing and enjoying the drive, Jo-Ann.

Thanks, Percy. I really appreciate this.

I'm glad that we're both relaxed, but please, be careful of what you eat, Jo-Ann.

Thanks for the reminder, Percy. You're my first priority. In fact, you are always on my mind. I'm careful of what I eat. I try to not become over excited. I check your equipment all of the time. I empty your bag as required. I mark my calendar and count the days for any one flange and bag we're wearing and change the full equipment as required. I dress for you, not necessarily for me. I walk each morning because I've realized this helps you function better. Sheesh, Percy. You're really high maintenance. Life with an ostomy always seems to be about input and output, whether we are at home or on the road.

I'm special.

Yes, you're special all right.

We arrived at our hotel and the celebration began. Son, Richard, our lovely daughter-in-law, Colleen, and our grandson, Evan, were in the room next to us. What a hoot! Daughter, Meredith, and her husband, James, arrived from Los Angeles. Oh, what fun. After a quick check on Percy, it was time to head off to Mono where we all got busy setting up and decorating the wedding facilities.

Setting up was very physical and I found that within about an hour, I was running out of steam. Percy had become very quiet — which I was grateful to my little buddy for. I switched my volunteer activities to kitchen duty where I could sit down while assisting in preparing food. This was helpful for me.

Later in the evening, when the hall was decorated and the food was prepared and stowed away in the refrigerators, it was time for the wedding rehearsal. By this time, I must admit I was in a bit of a foggy exhaustion as the rest of the family and friends revelled. Mark and his children are musicians, and so Percy and I sat down, I closed my eyes, and let the music of my beautiful blended family fill my heart.

When we arrived back at the hotel, which was about a thirty-minute drive, I was completely exhausted as I tumbled into bed and I fell asleep almost immediately. The thought on my mind was that Percy would stay quiet for the night and I could get a full night's sleep. Percy co-operated and I woke up feeling refreshed the following morning.

After a shower, breakfast, and attending to Percy's needs, it was time to dress for the wedding. I carefully unpacked Percy's new dress and wondered if it would fit well. I had lost a lot of weight after the surgery and my abdominal profile had changed now that the parastomal hernia was history. I lifted the dress over my head and put it on. Mark zipped the zipper and with a bit of apprehension I glanced at myself in the mirror.

Jo-Ann! The dress is stunning on us!

Yes, Percy. I'm so happy. too. Thank you again, Nola and the ladies at the dress shop. We did good.

Now time to head off to the wedding and celebrate Beth and Chris.

The wedding was beautiful and as with every wedding, there were some amazingly special moments. Beth and Chris were married outside in a gazebo. As Beth walked down the grassy hill wearing the wedding dress she had designed and sewed herself, two eagles soared and circled above us. Their graceful flight awed me. Then, as Beth and Chris stood together sharing their vows, several dragonflies appeared flying over their heads, ascending and simultaneously descending in a vortex of concentric circles. Wow. What gifts from Mother Earth for our two nature lovers.

We celebrated all day and well into the night, truly a day to remember. I'm so glad I am alive and well enough to share in this wonderful day. May Chris and Beth have a healthy, long, happy and prosperous life together.

The following day we all met for brunch. Thankfully, Percy had been quiet for the past couple of days, and well, it was time he woke up and he did. Before I could leave the restaurant, Percy started. Oh, dear. Percy was filling his bags as quickly as I could change them. How on earth am I going to be able to sit in a car for two hours with Percy emptying our whole bowel system? In and out of the bathroom I went, attending to Percy between eating toast and chitchatting with our children. Most interesting indeed. Oh, the life of an ostomate.

Sorry, but when nature calls ... Well ... You know.

I get it, Percy. All I can say right now is, I sure got my exercise!

With Percy finally settled down, it was in the car with us, and we were on our way to Lynn's home. When we arrived, my dear friend was waiting for us, she smiled and gave me a big hello. Wow. Her beautiful smile again captivated my heart. Forty years had gone by and her smile still glowed. I once again felt such love for my best friend and joy to be reunited.

Mark and Lynn hit it off right away and the three of us enjoyed our days visiting the many pretty and quaint Ontario towns along Lake Huron. Lynn prepared fantastic meals using local produce and introduced us to some of her friends. We dined in local restaurants, cooled ourselves at local pubs, and in the evening enjoyed comedy videos as we laughed and played together. We had a wonderful visit, and now it was time to head back home.

We split the trip into two sections for our drive so as to accommodate my healing body. We drove for about three hours to the home of son, Noah, his wife, Selina, and little granddaughter, Charlie. We spent the night enjoying each other then it was on the road again for another four-hour drive to our home. When we opened the door to our home, I was enchanted with our holiday away that had proven that Percy and I are now ready to get on with more spectacular recovery and life adventures.

6.4 Beyond Survival To Flourish

Filled with family and friends, our first road trip post surgery went very well.

We can do it, Percy!

We sure can.

I notice something, Jo-Ann.

You do? And what is that, Percy?

Well ... We're sitting outside in the back yard and all you have been doing is just sitting here. Once in a while you smile when a bird chirps, and you seem to be fascinated with the colour of the purple petunias in the hanging basket. Nothing else has entered your mind. It's so serene from where I am right now.

My gosh, Percy. You're right! Thanks for pointing this out to me. It's as though for the first time in at least six years that my mind and body isn't striving to deal with pain, cope with suffering, lift my spirits, or feel fuzzy from pain-management medications.

Although I was unwell for many years dealing with my bowel disorders, it was in 2008 when everything started coming apart. The beginning of the decline for me was 2008, and it was really and truly a battle that I was losing physically and emotionally. In retrospect, there is a degree of beauty in the failure of my body, and of the medical professionals at the time who were seemingly unable to properly diagnose me for so long, and which led to multiple hospital emergencies, then eventually to near death and life-saving surgery. All of which was followed by a long and often arduous recovery that included a second major surgery. I really feel, that back then, although I was stuck in a quagmire of pain, illness and desperation, the beauty of the journey of failures that filled and surrounded me was tangible and amazing. Don't get me wrong, during those years it was hard for me to see the forest for the trees while I was in the thick of things. And I was frustrated that all the plans I had made prior to my health decline had come undone.

The beauty that filled me was the realization that although I was immersed in adversarial circumstances and situations, I found out what I am capable of and what I can achieve when I put my mind, body, emotions and human spirit into it. The grand understanding is that not only do I possess many innate talents, skills, and abilities, I can also, when the need arises, become aware of them and in addition, I have an open mind for learning what I need to in order to create meaningful success for myself and my life, come what may. I realized, that in order to achieve any success I am reaching for, I must first be aware of and accept that every thought, emotion and action is motivated by conscious purpose. With a little luck sprinkled in, there is purpose in success.

The darkest of times brought me back and inspired me again along with the wisdom of the amazing women who are my grandmothers and my mother. I was transported back in time to the brilliance of a little boy, who is my son, Richard. Through every failure, these rivulets of ineffable wisdom flowed through my thoughts and experience. Every protective layer I had constructed in my mind and with my emotions, peeled back and the path to my authentic self, in all of its simplicity and complexity, was unearthed.

The beauty of my failures gave me the power to awaken and become more present in my life. The beauty did not stop there. I became filled with a transformative power that fuelled my perception of my self and of my life. Although life was surely slipping away from me, my failures provided me with the sustenance I needed to strive to survive while my whole self and life were in transition physically, emotionally, mentally and in spirit. So many times it was difficult to even imagine what was around the corner for me. I barely knew the right questions to ask or the best adjustments to make. The experience could lead me in different directions: I could succumb to anxiety and be over whelmed, or I could rise to the occasion with a good attitude peppered with courage.

My failure consisted of illness and pain that had become chronic. There were times when I was only able to take life one day at a time. Over time, I was eventually reduced to coping with my body and life one moment at a time. My failure found me searching, trying to find any reason, or any excuse, to have a positive outlook. Positive thoughts have their place in our lives, that is for certain, but to be honest, I could not go forward on positive thoughts alone. In fact, I realized this was not being totally honest with myself in thinking I was being positive while knowing in my heart that I was downright miserable, and terribly frightened. I was being drawn deeper and deeper into a physical, emotional, and mental bog. I was sick, angry, and fighting for my life, let alone struggling for quality of life.

Eventually, as the illness progressed, I arrived at the realization that I was taking life one breath at a time. It was becoming more and more challenging to remain honestly positive. My failure caused me to look the monster of my illness and my predicament in the eye with full awareness. This honest awareness empowered my human spirit. The only thing that was true to me at that time was that the "now", the "present", was the only reality that existed. I realized it was up to me to put as much into and receive as much as possible from each breath, that moment, that day. I was hurting in all ways possible so it was hard to see a positive future, but it was easy for me to immerse into my breath and explore the depths, wonders, and potentials that a breath can hold. I wore my string of breaths like a strand of pearls that encircled me with the hope and strength that life — at least for the moment — continued. I knew I would either live or I would die, but I sure wasn't going to go to either of these, defeated in spirit.

Success takes a lot of hard work and there must be purpose to that hard work. After the death of my late husband, Robert, a number of years ago, after thirty years of marriage, I had found myself having to build a new me, a new normal. As I sit here today, I now realize I've had a lot of experience with major life challenges. At any rate, I was required to take a long hard look at myself, my life and my future, as I was immersed in the grieving process. During that part of my experience, I realized that I was on a remarkable journey that was my life. I, like everyone on this planet, have developed talents, skills, abilities, individuality, and life strategies. These are tools we put into our personal and professional toolbox. As the events of my life unfold, when I need a particular tool or tools, I reach in and pull out the one that will work for me. I call this "self-coaching". Self-coaching is an ongoing process that I realize is a continual endeavour that assists us in being and doing all that we can be and do, to attain what we set out to gain and achieve. There is no doubt that the experiences of a present life is our blessing and our challenge. They are the facts of our lives. Within our inner reality we possess a universe of potential. Beyond ourselves there is also a universe of potentials. The illness I was experiencing helped me grow familiar with my inner spaces and how I connect with the outer expanses. I wanted to be successful at giving myself every chance for survival with quality of life. In the event survival was not to be for me, I would live what time I had left knowing the triumph of the human spirit. It has been a lot of hard work, it has been purposeful, and the challenge of success has been the most thrilling journey of a lifetime.

As Percy pointed out, in spite of it all and come what may, I have now arrived at the point whereby I am far and beyond basic survival and I am flourishing. Although I continue to live with the ravages left from the original disease, some complications from the extensive surgery, the ongoing everyday physical realities of living without part of my large bowel, and with Percy, my life has been forever changed. My foot is still dropping — not so much now, only when I'm tired — I have to attend to the psoriasis on my feet and heels, but I have for the time being, achieved serenity. I don't think I set out to achieve peace of mind, but I feel it is a by-product of the beauty of failure and the purpose of success.

6.5 Harmony and Celebration

As soon as we arrived home from our road trip, an email message arrived for us. A group called Author Land requested an interview for, *Better WITH a Bag than IN a Bag*". We were excited. This was our first literary interview on the book. Within a couple of days, *Better WITH a Bag than IN a Bag* reached #10 on the Indie Author Land Chart for summer reads. We were overjoyed. During this time, copies of the book were available to Kindle, Kobo and iTunes, and were selling in many countries. The feedback was very positive.

Percy and I have continued with writing and posting in *The Ostomy Factor* blog, which has attracted many folks from around the world, some of whom have become our friends. As we flourish, we are planning many other ostomy literary and speaking endeavours, and ostomy-related projects with the purpose of sharing, informing, and encouraging people who are having or have had ostomy surgery, and for their friends, family and medical professionals.

Party time, Jo-Ann!

Party time? Well yes. It sure is wonderful to be experiencing so much harmony at this time. It's a good reason to party.

I agree, Jo-Ann. But come on, don't you remember? It's time to celebrate.

And what are you so excited about?

In two days it'll be our second stomaversary!

Oh, goodness. That's right. Wow. Two years we've been together, little buddy.

Yup. So what do you have planned?

First, I have some glittery plastic jewels we will affix to your bag. You'll be covered with colourful bling. Then I think a night out on the town with Mark would be great. What do think of that, little buddy?

Sounds like a celebration to me.

And so, Percy was all aglow as we went to the Mooney's Bay Bistro for an evening of good eats, and we danced to the music of Johnny Vegas, with Eddie Bimm on the piano. It was a dreamy night with my two loves, Percy and Mark, and when we arrived back home later in the evening, we took a few moments to stand quietly in the back yard and we gazed at the stars.

It was a clear summer's eve as we stood holding hands looking up to the celestial marvel that graces our night sky. There were no shooting stars to make a wish upon. Instead, I thanked my lucky stars that I was still alive that night and that we were sharing our stomaversary together. We stood motionless as we witnessed the immensity and beauty of the Universe's starry realms. We opened our minds and bodies to the restless and dynamic cosmic power that is consistently constructing itself. I realized in that moment, like the Universe around me, all of us, no matter who we are, are masterpieces of humanity consistently sculpting our sense of self and designing our lives to fit the life and world around us.

Jo-Ann.

Yes, my Percy.

Just a few years ago the odds on you surviving were pretty low. With a lot of hard work, some luck, and the support of Mark and the family, look at you now! We've come a long way and we have a whole second lifetime ahead of us. Come what may, I'm with you all the way. We have so many adventures and special moments to experience. Life goes on.

Aww. Thank you. Life does go on, and so, another bag ... another day for us, little buddy.

One more request, Jo-Ann.

What's that?

I'd like to finish with a joke.

Take it away, Percy.

Knock, knock.
Who's there?

Stoma.
Stoma who?
The Stomamaster, Aha. I poop in our pouch without an ouch!

Epilogue

Another surgery is behind us. Now it's another bag, another day, and each day is a gift.

It's July 22, 2013, the day after our second stomaversary, our Celebration of Life Day was a success. It was a grand day filled with life, music, my loves, and stars to wish upon. For the past year, we got up and stepped out into a new life, a new world. At times, it was a struggle, at other times, Percy and I simply surrendered. For certain, though, at all times it was a marvellous exploration into the depths of ourselves and our lives as we endeavoured to bring out the best of who we are and share our journey with others.

Percy and I enjoyed writing this book together and so we have begun our next literary project that promises to be just as informative, inspiring and humorous. For up-to-date announcements and publishing dates, Google The Ostomy Factor and enter your email address to follow the blog and receive notifications of new posts by email. Don't be shy. Leave a comment or a review of the book. We love your feedback. And so, as Percy lies back in his hammock, and I get on with getting on with, thank you for marching forward with us to the beat of the recovery drum on this challenging and remarkable journey called life.

Acknowledgements

Percy and I would like to start by expressing our gratitude to everyone who has supported us during our healing adventure. We were never alone. Thank you to all of you who shared in this journey with us.

Mark Henderson, my life partner for your belief in me, and amazing support. Thank you for you.

Richard Tremblay, my son, you are my rock.

Rebecca Auer, MD, Msc, FRCSC, Surgical Oncologist/ Scientist at the Ottawa Hospital-General Campus. Thank you for your professionalism, expertise, and wonderful bedside manner.

Nancy Philip, Dr. Auer's assistant, for your patience and dedication to your patients.

Dr. Onochie, Internal Medicine, for your professional expertise, relentless pursuit for definitive diagnosis, and for your compassionate medical support.

Ottawa Hospital-General Campus, and floor nurses team and support staff. Thank you for your gentle administrations.

The Ontario Home Care Nurses. You are resourceful professionals with that personal touch.

Dr. Sarah Cohen DC, B.Sc. HK, SFR. DYNAMIC — optimizing *your health together.* Thank you for getting Percy and me in tip top shape. http://dynamicottawa.ca

Meredith Henderson, producer, editor, writer, actress; Sisbro & Co., Inc. Los Angeles, United States — media production including commercials, music videos, promos, film, TV and corporate videos. Thank you for your amazing creativity and media wizardry. www.sisbroandcompany.com

Crowe Creations, Sherrill Wark, editor — Thank you for ensuring this book made its way to publication with all the t's crossed and the i's dotted. Your support is so greatly appreciated. http://www.crowecreations.ca
.

Information, Tips & Hints

Suggested Valuable and Informative Ostomy-Related Websites:

Ostomy Canada Society Inc. (and in French, it is Société Canadienne des Personnes Stomisées). http://www.ostomycanada.ca

Ostomy Canada Society welcomes people, offering help and support to ostomates, their family, caregivers and friends. This website presents: support group local Chapter listings, connections to social media, Frequently Asked Questions (FAQ), and more information important to ostomates. In addition there is the "Ask the Ostomy Lifestyle Experts" section, information on manufacturers, links, publications and a blog.

A Guide to Living with a Stoma, http://www.living-with-a-stoma.co.uk and the sister website, *A Guide to Living with a Stoma, More for You*, http://www.livingwithastoma.co.uk

A Guide to Living with a Stoma and *A Guide to Living with a Stoma, More For You* are fun websites that offer comprehensive information on stoma lifestyle issues — at home, diet, on holiday and out and about. There are additional sections for accessories, blogs, books, events, foreign phrases, forums, magazines, new products, news, open days, ostomy glossary, paediatric, poems, songs, UK and worldwide suppliers and support organizations, and much more.

United Ostomy Association of America (UOAA), http://www.ostomy.org

This website presents information, help and support for people with an ostomy. It provides information about ostomies; answers questions about nutrition and intimacy; and provides useful knowledge about being an ostomate. The website states over 1,000,000 Americans have an ostomy, and over 130,000 new life-saving ostomy surgeries occur in America yearly, at the time of this printing. The United Ostomy Association of America is over 325 affiliated support groups strong. This association advocates for ostomates and their caregivers.

Global Associations

International Ostomy Association

http://www.ostomyinternational.org

An Association of Ostomy Associations, created to improve the life of ostomates worldwide. (Asia and South Pacific

Region, European Region, African Region, Ostomy Associations of Americas Region)

Ostomy Canada Society

http://www.ostomycanada.ca

United Ostomy Associations of America (UOAA)

http://www.ostomy.org/Home.html

Australian Council of Stoma Associations Inc.

http://www.australianstoma.com.au

Association Latino Americana de Ostomizados (South American Ostomy Association)

http://www.ostomyinternational.org/ALADO.htm

South African Stomal Therapy Association

http://www.stoma.co.za

Prolapse Stoma

A prolapse of the stoma occurs when the bowel protrudes through the stomal opening in the skin to a greater extent than was anticipated. The severity of the prolapse can vary from a small 2-3 centimetres (0.5 to 1 inch) to a large 10 centimetres (approximately 4 inches). Any prolapse is frightening and distressing for the patient and should be handled sensitively.

Parastomal Hernias

What is a parastomal hernia?

When a person has a stoma it can develop into an ostomy-specific type of hernia called a parastomal hernia. Since a stoma passes through the abdomen, it can compromise the strength of the muscular abdominal wall. These weakened muscles can come away from the stoma, weakening its integrity and causing the intestine to bulge.

A stoma hernia can be uncomfortable and unnerving, not to mention more difficult to manage and care for. As the abdominal profile grows, it can become more difficult to attach ostomy equipment. It can also eventually lead to intestinal twisting/kinking that can cause serious damage to the intestine by cutting off blood vessels. (If this happens, the ostomate must seek immediate medical attention as this condition being left untreated can be very dangerous.)

What causes a parastomal hernia?

Coughing, sneezing, heavy lifting, and anything that will put pressure on the abdominal wall and the stoma. Over time, muscles can weaken to the point that the stoma can begin to protrude and push out due to the pressure of the internal guts behind it. There are many possible origins for a parastomal hernia to develop. Some are related to surgery, a poorly placed stoma, or the developing of an infection around the border.

How is a parastomal hernia treated?

Surgery is the most common repair for any type of large hernia. Typically, ostomates are encouraged to wear a hernia belt before being recommended surgery. A hernia belt is a firm, wide belt that helps support the stoma and muscle tissue around it externally. When surgery is recommended, options will be considered and discussed. There are two options:

• To repair the muscle tissue around the stoma (either with stitching or mesh).

• Create a new opening in a healthy spot and close off the old one.

Drop Foot

Drop foot, or Foot Drop as it may also be called, refers to a weakening of the muscles that allow one to flex the ankle and toes, causing the individual to drag the front of the foot while walking, and to compensate for this scuffle by bending the knee to lift the foot higher than usual.

While drop foot is a neuromuscular disorder that affects the nerves and muscles, it is not actually a disease in itself but rather a symptom of some other medical problem, possibly by a condition in the low back.

Ostomy Equipment and Potential Leakage

Ostomy leakage is a problem that all ostomates will no doubt encounter at some point during their time with a stoma. For most people, it's a common occurrence in the early weeks of managing an ostomy when they are still finding their ostomy-feet and working out which products are best for them, and which routine gives the best results. It can cause a heck of a mess, not only to our clothes, but to our self-confidence, too.

To find out what is causing the leakage, start by checking the back of the flange after it's leaked and you've removed it. This holds the biggest clue of all. You will be able to see what path the stool took on its break to freedom. Compare this to your skin and see what problems are present.

1. Condition of the skin. Is it raw, or does it have a rash all over it, or on part of it? If so, you may be allergic to the flange, and it may be interfering with the adhesive properties of the flange. Also, check to see if the area around where the flange leaks is any worse than elsewhere.

2. With leakage, the stool will always follow the path of least resistance. Do you have a belly crease which in turn is

creasing the flange and creating a nice little tunnel for your stool to escape?

3. Look at your flange. Was the gap around the stoma too large? Or was it too tight? Or just right? Do you have protruding stitches around your stoma which the flange has trouble moulding around?

4. Do you have a belly cavity near the stoma? Flanges may struggle to adhere to these dips in your belly and lead to leakage.

5. Check your stoma. Is it flat/flush to the skin? Is it inverted/pulled in?

Some causes of leakage could be:

• Flush to the skin or inverted stoma

• Poor-fitting flange/odd shaped stoma

• Belly cavity around stoma

• Parastomal hernia and/or pancaking

Once you've discovered the source of your leakage, then you are in a better position to be successful in stopping your leakage in its tracks, and there are a number of products available on the market that are designed to help reduce opportunities for leakage to occur.

Arrange a visit with an enterostomal therapy nurse, (ET nurse — registered nurse (RN) who has specialized training in treating patients with ostomies), they can assist you in assessing the leakage issue and make equipment product recommendations for ensuring a good seal. One thing to bear in mind with all ostomy products is that our bodies are very individual, and because of that, a product which works great for one person may not work anywhere near as successfully for another, and vice versa. You may need to sample various rings and seals to find the one that works best for you, which all of the various ostomy product companies will assist you in finding the seal that will work for you. So there is no reason why you cannot use multiple products to help combat leakage.

Stigma

I feel, to better understand "stigma", as it relates to ostomates, I will share an article I wrote that was published in *Ostomy Canada* Magazine (Summer 2015 Edition).

The Long, Slow Battle: How we can rise above stigma — By Jo-Ann L. Tremblay

A gentleman (ostomy 5 years) in the United States, registered to join an aqua fitness program at a local recreation facility pool. Upon learning of his ostomy, the program director attempted to persuade him to locate and join another fitness program, instead.

A woman (ileostomy 25 years) in the United Kingdom, has four adult children, and she hasn't told them about her ostomy. She feels people should not talk about it, and that there will always be a stigma attached.

A young man (recent ostomy), in Canada, laments over the break up of his nine year relationship with as he describes, "the love of my life". His partner ended the relationship stating, "You're not attractive to me anymore, you've changed".

A wife concerned for her husband, (ostomy three years), who had battled colon cancer, is now cancer free and has a permanent ostomy. He won't go out, he won't travel anymore, and he has stopped visiting friends. His wife wants to know how she can help him feel better about himself.

These are just four of the many overt and subtle stigma related stories people have shared with me. To better understand what is happening with and to ostomates, we should have a basic understanding of what stigma is, where it comes from, its impacts, and how we can make a difference.

Online dictionary meanings for stigma are:

- *a disgusting mark or social disgrace*
- *a stain or reproach, as on one's reputation*
- *a mark or obvious trait that is characteristic*
- *a defect or disease*

When a body is impaired in some way, including the creation of an ostomy, many people experience emotional and psychological distress. Depending on the original disease and treatment that required the creation of the ostomy most people probably spent quite a lot of time in private and public restroom facilities, which was likely embarrassing to them. For some, this may have been the time when the seed of stigmatization was planted.

On an ongoing basis, ostomates have many challenges to content with. Daily, we must attend to the basic physical maintenance related to our ostomy, and this is just the beginning. We are required to deal with the psychological impacts our ostomy has on our social and family relationships, travel, nutrition, physical activity, sexual function, economic issues, and more ...

We must consistently observe our parastomal skin, and then do our best to stave off skin irritations and rashes. Due to incontinence we feel a loss of control, which causes many of us to experience sleep disturbances, and of course there are the occasional uncontrolled gas emissions in the presence of others. Although the various ostomy equipment companies manufacture high quality products, leakage accidents happen which, of course is very disconcerting. All of this worry has an effect on our quality of life and attitude towards ourselves.

Our ostomies are a mixed blessing, on one hand they are the medical miracles that give us a second chance at life for wellness, energy and the opportunity to live life to the fullest, come what may. An ostomy is also a constant reminder of the illness we experienced, and the damage it caused. There are a wide range of quality of life issues that challenge and impact ostomates.

Society places a great deal of emphasis on body image. Then, there are the potty training experiences we endured as children. The things that happen during potty training will stay with us forever. For example: how it is a horrible thing to have an accident, or becoming intolerant of those who have medical problems that cause incontinence.

All of these factors fuel stigmatization from others, and the self-stigmatization some ostomates experience. The worst part of stigma is that people often internalize feelings of shame and it becomes a vicious cycle, a cycle whereby every new attack makes the victim more vulnerable to further stigma abuse.

How do we rise above stigma? Beginning with self-stigmatization, we can, one step at a time, turn this around by accepting the changes and transitions we experience through our attitude. Even if it is baby steps, they are still steps. A positive attitude truly helps us transform and settle into our new normal. We know of course this is more easily said than done, but the effort is well worth it. It really does pay off in the long run.

Scientific research states, when we think positive thoughts the brain releases endorphins, while negative thoughts release chemicals recorded during depression episodes. Now of course positive thinking alone will most probably not pull someone out of a major depressed state. But, we can give ourselves a daily dose of positive thinking and the attendant endorphins will happen naturally. This certainly can help get us through a lot of stress.

We have our own free will, and we are responsible for building upon our individual positive attitude. Having said this, one of the greatest of gifts others can give that will help us to accept our body and new normal is to know people care. Some of us may have a partner or support person who can inspire us to accept ourselves. For some, friends and family are not equipped to provide it. Whatever the case may be for you, you're not alone. Endeavour to search out and connect with your local/national Ostomy Support Groups, read ostomy related books, and join on-line groups/forums. These groups and activities are designed and intended to provide positive energy, valuable suggestions based on experience, and support.

If you encounter someone who is stigmatizing you, know they are misinformed. A terrible part of stigma is that the victim often internalizes the feelings these sweeping judgements can cause. As human beings we are acutely responsive to how other people perceive, evaluate, and feel about us individually. We are attuned to others' reactions to us, and if we perceive other people are interested, approving, or accepting of us, over time the positive responses from those folks will foster psychological and physical well-being. If we perceive that others are disinterested, disapproving or rejecting, over a long-term this exposure to the negative interpersonal reactions will then cause us psychological difficulties and potential poor physical health. Basically, other people's reactions exert a strong impact on our thoughts, emotions, motives, and behaviour, as well as our physical and psychological well-being. If a person overtly or subtly stigmatizes you, (for example — implies your original illness and resultant ostomy is due to a personal sickness, saying "it's your fault, you got sick," you may want to open up to help educate them).

Your willingness to share your story can really make a difference. Opening up helps educate others, the more people who know about an ostomy, and ostomates living a full life, in spite of it all, the less likely they are to stigmatize. Everyone you meet has a story to tell, and when you know someone's story, it's much harder to make negative generalizations.

Keeping your ostomy a secret can be isolating, and going public can be overwhelming to be sure, but it's a way you can rise above stigma, misconceptions and prejudice, to show others that they are not so different from you and me.

A few months ago I experienced a subtle form of stigma when I attended my arts group, "Share Your Art" event. I proudly placed "Percy a Self Portrait" on the easel. I looked out to the audience, and then began to explain that the piece of art is an oil on canvas painting, and I shared a brief back story. I explained the portrait subject matter is a stoma, an ostomy flange, and a partial abdomen. Almost instantly, the faces of many of my fellow artists showed a reaction. I noticed some eyebrows lowered, some noses wrinkled, and many lips became pressed together. It is important to note that not all of the audience members had a look of disgust on their faces. I continued with my presentation by informing them that a stoma is often referred to as a rose bud. I then turned the picture upside down and voila the audience saw a beautiful rosebud instead of a stoma. There was an almost immediate change of expression on the faces of most of the audience members. Some faces now had a look of pleasure, some a look of relief, others of admiration, and there was a sprinkle of nervous laughs that rippled through the room. Interesting, it was the same picture, only the orientation was different.

By the way, the ostomate in the US who was being encouraged to find another aqua fitness program, met with his local ostomy support group. *It was decided that three of the support group members and the gentleman himself would meet with the aqua fitness program director to educate her on what an ostomy is and how it is managed. When she had a better understanding, she welcomed the ostomate, and he's now enjoying the fitness improvement and social aspects the program offers.*

The woman in the UK still has not talked with her adult children about her ileostomy, and does not intend to.

The young Canadian man is working on the understanding that some people just don't cope well with what they perceive as a defect, and is pleased to share that he is building on his personal self-esteem. He has joined an ostomy dating and social network group.

As his partner and supporter, the wife of the almost-shut-in ostomate is intent on inspiring her husband by setting a positive tone with the idea of helping him cope with his transition and change. She is working on noticing the potential benefits of his ostomy, while accepting his pain, and is taking the appropriate opportunities to share her observations with him. She accepts his ostomy as a natural part of his body. This is helping him to accept it as his new normal. She perceives him as a whole person. This is helping him feel intact. And finally, she stays open to the potential that there will be people who are not able to join her and her husband in accepting the change, and will deal with this if and when it arises.

It is important to know that vulnerable victims of stigma, whether it is self-inflicted or forced upon them by others, are all experiencing isolation, loneliness and interpersonal rejection. Ostomates have already endured a terrible illness and the journey that brought them to the creation of their ostomy. It's our second chance at life to live it to the fullest in spite of it all. What a shame, that an ostomate must also then suffer stigma. Although we know social and cultural shifts are a long and slow battle, we can rise above stigma by being a source of support for each other. Through our individual and collective efforts, we can foster acceptance of our own ostomy, and on behalf of our fellow ostomates. By being active advocates and educators, we can change perceptions. When we step forward with our stories and live by example, with a bit of time and effort, we will transcend the limitations of stigma to make a difference.

Emptying Your Ostomy Pouch

Emptying your ostomy pouch seems to be an individual thing. Whatever way you have discovered, it's okay. You do have a few options when emptying your pouch at home:

• You can sit far back on the toilet seat.

• Kneel on the floor beside the toilet. (Use a towel or pillow to protect your knees.)

• You can stand over the toilet.

• You can sit on the side.

• You can sit on a stool beside the toilet.

Whatever position you choose that is proper for you, will work. If you opt for a stool beside the toilet, there are a few important measurements you will want to keep in mind.

Research results reveal the height of traditional toilets will vary from 35 cm (14 inches), to 43 cm (17 inches). Sometimes an individual needs a little assistance, and so the disability access toilets and models comfortable for seniors are usually about 5.08 cm (2 inches) taller than the traditional models. For these folks, the added height can make a difference when it comes to sense of ease and everyday comfort. So it is recommended that before you purchase a stool, make sure you've measured your toilet height, and buy the stool that matches that height.

- Sit far back on the seat, sit on the side, use a stool, kneel on the floor or stand over the toilet.

- Make sure to have a piece of toilet paper within reach.

- Raise the pouch so the opening faces up.

- Open the pouch. You will unclamp or unroll the integrated drainage outlet.

- Lower the opening into the toilet. Slide your hands down the pouch to push out the stool.

- If you stand while emptying the pouch, you may want to flush the toilet as you drain the pouch or place a few pieces of toilet paper into the toilet bowl. This prevents the stool and toilet water from splashing up when draining from high distance.

- Wipe the opening off inside and out with toilet paper or tissue.

- If used, add pouch deodorant at this time.

• Re-clamp or reseal the pouch.

Emptying Your Pouch When You're Out

To be sure, emptying an ostomy pouch can be difficult in some public washroom facilities; however, this is a problem that a person encounters with or without a stoma. If you usually empty your pouch by sitting on the toilet seat in a position that you can empty the pouch between your legs into the commode, for example, sitting on the public toilet seat is a challenge when the facilities are not clean. This is when you adapt your pouch-emptying procedure to best suit the circumstances. You can opt to stand in front of or beside the toilet, lean forward and empty the pouch. You'll want to roll down the integrated drainage outlet or remove the clip carefully, aim the end of the pouch into the toilet and empty. Wipe off the end of the pouch with toilet paper. Refasten with the clip or roll up the drainage outlet and presto, you're done! Ensure if you use a clip that you keep it out of harm's way when emptying your pouch. Always carry a spare pouch clip with you when you will be emptying away from home or are travelling. Take your time when refastening the pouch clip as you may be more apt to fumble the clip into the toilet when you are in hurry.

Sharing Ostomy Fashion Ideas

Where your stoma is located will have a big impact on how you wear clothes. Because stoma placement differs from person to person, some adjustments are needed. I found, initially, when my stoma was first created, that when I wore clothes with a waistband, it was a challenge. Four years later, it is only at times that waistbands and clothes with zippers can be annoying and uncomfortable for me. In speaking with my fellow ostomates at our Ostomy Canada Society Chapter, the following are a few of their suggestions for your information and experimentation.

- There are many reputable companies that manufacture clothing for ostomates. You may want to explore. You can Google — ostomy garments, ostomy swimsuits, etc.

- Visit some of your local maternity shops. They can offer some pieces of leisure clothing that you might find comfortable.

- Ostomy support wraps/maternity bands. These pieces of clothing can range from basic maternity wraps to more specialty wraps made for ostomates. They allow for the concealment of your appliance, and offer some support, too. Wraps designed for ostomates usually have pockets which you can fit your pouch into. This helps to keep the bottom of the pouch from hanging below the bottom of the wrap.

- Pouch Covers. Pouch covers are made to hide the contents of your pouch (when using a transparent pouch). They have many patterns, styles and materials available.

- High-waisted pants/undergarments. There are high-waisted products which are designed specifically for ostomates. Also, you can find high-waisted products in most clothing stores. Your goal here is to keep your pouch below the belt line without the need for any other accessories. Many ostomy high-waisted products offer security pouch pockets.

- Stoma guards. Stoma guards can be extremely useful if your stoma is at, or above, your belt line. They offer men and women protection from impact, seat belts or pant belts, and they'll often allow you to wear your pouch inside your slacks with your blouse tucked in. Men can wear their pouch inside their pants with their shirt tucked in. (Depending on the style of your stoma guard, output is usually not restricted, however pouch capacity can be reduced.)

- Stealth Belt. The Stealth Belt allows you to wear your pouch horizontally. There are many styles you can research that may work for you.

Casual Clothing: For the ladies and the gentlemen, dressing casual is one of the easiest ways to dress with an ostomy. Since with casual clothing we can leave blouses and shirts untucked, and they are often loose-fitting, there is less need to worry about concealing or protecting your stoma and equipment. When at home, some folks have suggested that they leave their pouch over their slacks/pants and let their shirt cover it. Of course track pants, stretch pants and sweatpants are also options. Clothing with elastic waists often accommodate most stoma placements.

When going out, some folks put a wrap on, which offers a low profile. It is suggested that jeans shouldn't be tight, and it is highly recommended getting a pair that have some stretch to the denim, especially if the pouch will be tucked into your slacks.

Semi-casual/Semi-Formal: The ladies can wear dresses, many styles are comfortable. Skirts with a high waist work well. You can wear a nice wrap or jacket to spruce up the dress. For the gentlemen, semi-casual means they can leave a shirt untucked. The fellas can wear a stoma guard. If the stoma is above the belt line often the pouch under the belt is restrictive and may cut off the flow of output. Some guards correct the problem by channelling output to flow down to the bottom of the pouch, without being restricted or cut off by the belt.

Formal: Again, the ladies can wear comfortable dresses. Like semi-casual, the men often want to wear their shirt tucked in. It's suggested that they'll want to apply the same methods when wearing semi-casual clothing. Methods such as: stoma guard, a stealth belt, and/or suspenders when necessary. High-waisted option or elastic waist bands are comfortable. The goal here is to comfortably tuck your ostomy appliance under your dress or pants.

In conclusion, the most important thing you need, is to be comfortable. Often ostomates feel the ostomy equipment attached to them is obvious. When we look in the mirror, we notice the equipment under our clothes. It's agreed by many ostomates that most people won't notice our ostomy. Many ostomates shared with me that they got used to their ostomy, and they figured out tips and tricks for feeling comfortable, and if it is important to them, keeping their ostomy equipment concealed.

.

About the Author

Jo-Ann L. Tremblay is a personal/professional life coach, trainer, photographer, and water colour/oil artist. This is her third book. Her other books include *Better WITH a Bag than IN a Bag — From the brink of death to recovery through humour and inspiration*, and *The Self-Coaching Toolbox — Six tools for personal and professional growth & development,* soon to be available in a revised edition. In support of her awareness and advocacy 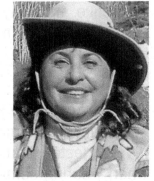 endeavours, Jo-Ann is a blogger of *The Ostomy Factor*. Jo-Ann has created and hosted the television special, *That's Life*, hosted two television program series — and a radio program series, *Voices of Our Town*.

After a lengthy illness, Jo-Ann underwent life-saving surgery that resulted in the creation of an ostomy and the stoma she affectionately calls "Percy". Now an ostomate, Jo-Ann L. Tremblay joins with fellow ostomates, their caregivers, medical experts and people in general, through speaking engagements, writing magazine articles, and is a member of the Medical Advisory Committee in the capacity of Ostomy Lifestyle Expert with the Canada Ostomy Society.

Website: www.jo-annltremblay.com
Blog: joannltremblay.wordpress.com *(The Ostomy Factor)*
Twitter: @joanntremblay
Facebook: Author Jo-Ann L. Tremblay

Other Books by Jo-Ann L. Tremblay

Better WITH a Bag Than IN a Bag

ISBN-13: 978-0-9809009-1-0

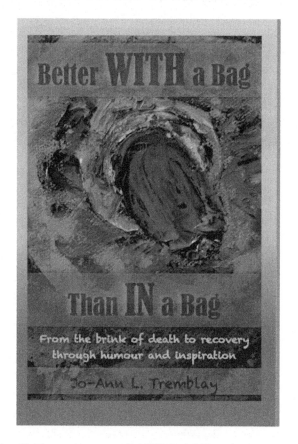

Available on Amazon (PAPERBACK and KINDLE),
throughout the world

As an E-BOOK on iTunes
As an E-BOOK on Kobo

In PAPERBACK at:
Barnes and Noble   Alibris.com or Alibris UK

The Self-Coaching Toolbox
(Original Paperback Edition)

ISBN 1-897113-06-4

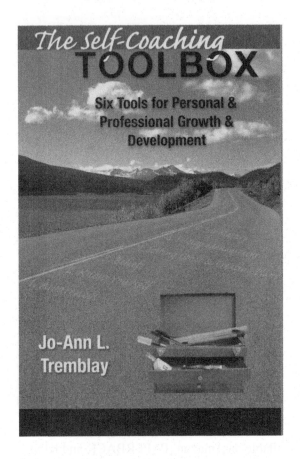

Available for purchase at
www.amazon.com